AF872251

Attention-Based Machine Learning for Diabetes Mellitus Risk Assessment, Prediction, and Classification

Fabian

Table of contents

LIST OF TABLES

LIST OF FIGURES

LIST OF ABBREVIATIONS

DM	Diabetes Mellitus
DL	Deep Learning
ML	Machine Learning
LSTM	Long- And Short-Term Memory
DNN	Deep Neural Network
T1DM	Type-1 Diabetes Mellitus
T2DM	Type-2 Diabetes Mellitus
GDM	Gestational Diabetes Mellitus
PCOS	Polycystic Ovary Syndrome
MODY	Maturity-Onset Diabetes Of The Young
NDM	Neonatal Diabetes Mellitus
TNDM	Transient Neonatal Diabetes Mellitus
SVM	Support Vector Machines
SLFN	Single-Hidden-Layer Feedforward Networks
KNN	K-Nearest Neighbours
GBM	Gradient Boosting Machines
NB	Naive Bayes
CNN-LSTM	Convolutional Neural Network-Long Short Term Memory
CGM	Continuous Glucose Monitoring

PCA	Principal Components Analysis
RNN	Recurrent Neural Network
DNN	Deep Neural Network
IBESOA	Improved Bald Eagle Search Optimization Algorithm
Bi-LSTM-CNN	Bi-Directional-Long Short Term Memory- Convolutional Neural Network
CA-Bi-GRU	Correlation Attention-Based Bi-Directional Gate Recurrent Unit
TABO	Tunicate Assisted Butterfly Optimization
TSO	Tunicate Search Optimization
BOA	Butterfly Optimization Algorithm
ELM	Extreme Learning Model
Bi-GRU	Bi-Directional Gate Recurrent Unit
DT	Decision Tree
SVC	Support Vector Classification
XGB	Extreme Gradient Boosting
SHAP	Shapley Additive Explanations
R-SVM	Radial Support Vector Machine
TCN	Temporal Convolution Networks
ENN	Edited Nearest Neighbor
SMOTE-N	Synthetic Minority Over Sampling For Nominal Data

SMOTE-ENN	Synthetic Minority Over Sampling For Nominal- Edited Nearest Neighbor
NOD	New-Onset Diabetes
PDAC	Patients Developing Pancreatic Ductal Adenocarcinoma
SMBO	Sequential Model-Based Optimization
Att-Bi-LSTM-CNN	Attention-Based (Att) Bi-Directional Long-And Short-Term Memory-Convolutional Neural Network
CNN	Convolutional Neural Networks
FCL	Fully Connected Layer
MAR	Missing At Random
RFE	Recursive Feature Elimination
EAGA-MLP	Enhanced And Adaptive-Genetic Algorithm-Multilayer Perceptron
LIME	Local Interpretable Model-Agnostic Explanations,
(Grad-CAM)	Gradient-Weighted Class Activation Mapping
DFU	Diabetes Foot Ulcer
UNet-CRF-RNN	Unet-Conditional Random Field-Recurrent Neural Network

CHAPTER 1

INTRODUCTION

1.1. DIABETES MELLITUS

Diabetes Mellitus (DM) is a chronic metabolic disorder that gradually worsens and is characterized by high blood sugar levels that persist for a long time. The high blood sugar results from a lack of insulin, resistance to insulin, or a combination of both. According to the changes in lifestyle and the aging of the population due to the fast-globalizing world, diabetes has become the leading cause of global health challenges in the current century (Celli et al., 2022). Besides its metabolic perturbation, DM mellitus negatively affects different organ systems and is a major cause of disease, death, and decrease in quality of life all over the world. Hence, timely diagnosis, severity grading, and early treatment have become essential parts of healthcare systems nowadays(Alam et al., 2021) The word diabetes means excessive urination, and mellitus indicates the presence of glucose in the urine. DM develops due to impairment in secretion or action of insulin which leads to abnormal carbohydrate, protein, and lipid metabolism besides hyperglycaemia (Chaki et al., 2022). The long, term increase of blood glucose level may become more than the absorption capacity of the kidneys causing sugar to be excreted in the urine and excessive hunger and if the condition is left uncontrolled, it may cause diabetic retinopathy, neuropathy, nephropathy, cardiovascular diseases, as well as impaired wound healing mainly in the lower extremities which causes increased risk of gangrene and amputation(Md. J. Hossain et al., 2024) . Research shows that treatment of blood sugar levels, blood pressure, and following a good diet, being physically active and lifestyle modification will have significant effects in the prevention of these complications, (Osunde et al., 2025).

While tests like fasting plasma glucose, oral glucose tolerance tests, and glycated hemoglobin (HbA1c) are available to standardize biochemical diagnostics, the traditional diagnostic methods that are mostly used are still reactive and only show a static snapshot of metabolic status. These methods do not capture disease progression, inter, patient variability, and latent risk patterns, so diagnosis is often delayed and complication rates are higher. Diabetic retinopathy (DR), one of the most serious microvascular complications of diabetes and a major cause of vision loss, needs to be detected in time in order to be able to rescue the eye from irreversible damage.(Kropp et al., 2023) Although fundus examination with manual grading by ophthalmologists is the clinical gold standard, it is a very long process, subjective, and varies from one doctor to another, especially in the early stages of the disease. Even if the automation has been improved by recent deep learning, based methods, most of them use retinal images only, thus their diagnostic reliability is very low in visually ambiguous cases and they do not take into consideration the complementary clinical information (Sobhi et al., 2025).

Advances in medical science, the digital health infrastructure, and artificial intelligence have opened the doors to data, driven healthcare solutions. This is made possible by the increasing availability of electronic health records, continuous glucose monitoring systems, and large, scale clinical datasets. One significant development is the application of machine learning (ML) and deep learning (DL) algorithms to clinical decision, support systems, which has led to the early detection, personalized treatment, and improved disease surveillance. However, the prevalence of diabetes is increasing at an alarming rate. The widespread adoption of sedentary lifestyles, poor dietary habits, obesity, stress, and genetic predisposition are some of the factors causing this rise, especially in low, and middle, income countries (Sharif et al., 2023).

In India, diabetes has become a major health crisis that affects both urban and rural populations. The lack of early screening, limited follow, up, and shortage of individualized risk assessment tools are some of the factors that worsen disease outcomes in these areas. These problems point to the necessity of intelligent, scalable, affordable, and clinically interpretable diagnostic frameworks that can integrate retinal imaging with clinical and temporal data to provide proactive, precision, based diabetes management (Brar et al., 2022).

1.2. TYPES OF DM

DM is primarily classified into three main types:

1. Type 1DM (T1DM)
2. Type 2DM (T2DM)
3. Gestational DM (GDM)

1.2.1. T1DM

The hallmark of T1DM is a chronic autoimmune illness marked by loss of pancreatic beta cells producing insulin, characterized by an absolute lack of insulin. T1DM can appear at any age, in contrast to type 2 diabetes, which is primarily linked to insulin resistance (Karamanakos et al., 2022). T1DM typically first appears in childhood or adolescence. While the precise etiology of type 1 diabetes remains unclear, environmental factors and genetic predisposition are thought to play a combined role. The presence of certain diseases or environmental factors may induce an autoimmune response in a person who has a genetic predisposition to the illness (Khan et al., 2021). This indicates that the immune system of the individual will unintentionally target and kill the beta cells in the pancreas that make insulin. As a consequence of this autoimmune destruction, insulin, the hormone that regulates blood sugar levels, eventually becomes inadequate (Apostolopoulou et al., 2025).

Increased thirst, frequent urine, excessive appetite, polyphagia, fatigue, unexplained weight loss, and blurred eyesight are some of the features that characterize type 1 diabetes. In most cases, it will present with sudden symptoms. The rapid development of these symptoms over some days or weeks can be an indication of T1DM (Ortiz-Martínez et al., 2022) In case of improper timely treatment of T1DM with symptoms of high blood sugar levels and the presence of ketones building up in the blood, T1DM patients are prone to a potentially fatal sickness called diabetic ketoacidosis. The diagnosis of autoimmune T1DM may be strengthened by the discovery of autoantibodies (such as anti-GAD and anti-IA-2 antibodies) directed against pancreatic beta cells (Vargas et al., 2023).

When controlling T1DM, blood sugar levels must be maintained within a target range to prevent both short- and long-term complications. Type 1 diabetics cannot produce insulin on their own, hence exogenous insulin supplementation is necessary for survival. There are several different types of insulin formulations available, including short-, intermediate-, and rapid-acting. Insulin can be continuously or multiple times daily subcutaneously administered with insulin pumps (Thotad et al., 2023). Regular self-monitoring with a glucose meter is crucial for managing blood sugar levels and adjusting insulin dosage. Eating a balanced meal high in carbohydrates, proteins, and fats as well as routinely calculating carbohydrates can help people with T1DM better control their blood sugar levels. Regular exercise plays a major role in improving insulin sensitivity and overall health. To avoid hypo- or hyperglycemia, people with T1DM should check their blood sugar levels before, during, and after exercise (Rosengren & Dikaiou, 2023). Diabetes education initiatives offer important information about blood sugar monitoring, insulin delivery methods, self-management tactics, and identifying and handling hypo- and hyperglycemic episodes. It might be difficult to manage T1DM emotionally and physically. People's quality of life can be enhanced and their ability to manage the demands of their illness increased with the assistance of peers, family, and medical professionals (Jiang et al., 2023). Several acute and long-term problems, such as hypo or hyperglycemia, diabetic ketoacidosis (DKA), cardiovascular disease, neuropathy, nephropathy, retinopathy, and poor wound healing, can result from poorly managed type 1 diabetes. To avoid or postpone the beginning of these problems, strict glycemic management and routine medical follow-up are crucial (Prampolini et al., 2025)

1.2.2. T2DM

Type-2 diabetes is a long-term metabolic illness characterised by relative insulin insufficiency and resistance to its effects (Boye et al., 2022) It is the most common kind of diabetes, accounting for the vast majority of cases worldwide. Although more recently being diagnosed in children and adolescents, T2D generally occurs in adults. This is almost corroborated by an increased occurrence of obesity and sedentariness. A person with type 2 diabetes (T2D) develops resistance in their body to the effects of the pancreatic hormone insulin, which is involved in transferring glucose from the bloodstream into cells for energy (Y. Chen et al., 2023). This results in hyperglycemia and elevated blood glucose concentration. When the pancreas is finally unable to secrete enough insulin to overcome insulin resistance, then hyperglycemia can become worse. Obesity, physical inactivity, several variables, including genetic predisposition, aging, ethnicity, gestational diabetes, polycystic ovarian syndrome (PCOS), and certain drugs (such as corticosteroids and antipsychotics), can result in the development of type 2 diabetes (T2DM) (Suwarno, 2024). The onset of T2DM is often gradual, and many individuals may remain asymptomatic for years. On the other hand, some people could receive an unintentional diagnosis during regular medical exams. Oral glucose tolerance testing, fasting blood sugar measurements, or Measurements of the HbA1c level are frequently used in Type-2 diabetes. When blood sugar levels routinely surpass diagnostic thresholds, a diagnosis is verified (Hanna et al., 2023).

Glycemic control and improvement of insulin sensitivity can be achieved by a healthy diet, regular exercise, weight management, and stopping smoking.(Yefet et al., 2023) Treatment modality that involves dietary modification could be by way of regulation of processed foods loaded with sugar, monitoring carbohydrate intake, limiting portion sizes, and overall fiber-enriched diets. Some may need insulin therapy to attain good glycemic goals (Azmi et al., 2023a). Persons with T2D can monitor their progress, see trends, and modify the adjustments in self-management that they have made in their treatment plan by periodically self-monitoring with a blood glucose meter. Frequent medical check-ups are crucial for the early identification and treatment of issues related to T2D (Azmi et al., 2023b). Diabetes education initiatives offer important information on blood sugar monitoring, medication adherence, lifestyle changes, and self-management techniques. Diabetes educators, peer support groups, and healthcare practitioners can empower people with T2D to take charge of their health and make educated decisions(Ansari et al., 2024). Numerous acute and long-term problems, such as peripheral vascular disease, neuropathy, nephropathy, retinopathy, cardiovascular disease, and diabetic foot ulcers, can result from poorly managed T2D. For these problems to be prevented or postponed, strict glucose control, blood pressure management, and cholesterol control are necessary.

1.2.3. GDM

The second or third trimester of pregnancy is usually when GDM, a transient form of diabetes, first appears. Hyperglycaemia, or high blood sugar, is one of its hallmarks and can be dangerous for the foetus as well as the mother (Ahmed et al., 2023). The body's incapacity to generate adequate insulin during pregnancy leads to gestational diabetes mellitus(Mavroeidi et al., 2024). Hormonal changes in pregnancy could be responsible, including the effect of elevated progesterone, estrogen, and human placental lactogen, which may result in a condition called insulin resistance whereby body cells lose their sensitivity to insulin(X. Yu et al., 2023). Blood glucose levels will rise, giving way to GDM in the event that the pancreas cannot produce enough insulin to compensate. Women whose risks of developing GDM are high include those above 25 years, obese, with a family history of diabetes, a prior history of GDM, PCOS, Hispanic, African American, Asian origin, parity, and gestation period—late in pregnancy(Gautam et al., 2025). Screening for GDM is done using an oral glucose tolerance test approximately during weeks 24 and 28 of pregnancy. To diagnose GDM, a confirmatory OGTT is carried out if the findings of the first screening are abnormal(Wong & Sattar, 2023). Certain women can be more vulnerable and need to be screened earlier. Many women with GDM are detected through standard screening while they are asymptomatic. Nonetheless, certain individuals can encounter indications including heightened thirst, frequent urination, exhaustion, impaired vision, or recurring infections (Hong et al., 2022). Pre-eclampsia, caesarean delivery, and macrosomia (high birth weight) are among pregnancy issues that can result from GDM (Kieu et al., 2023).

Gestational DM management aims to minimize risks to both the mother and the foetus by achieving and sustaining healthy blood sugar levels. The diet should emphasize complex carbohydrates, lean protein, and healthy fat sources, and include an abundance of fruits and vegetables. Patients can be counselled to do carbohydrate counting and, if needed, portion control to help in maintaining normal postprandial glucose levels. Regular physical activity—brisk walking, swimming, or prenatal yoga, enhances insulin sensitivity and thus helps in blood sugar control. It is, however, always advisable to consult a doctor before commencing exercises on the course of pregnancy. Otherwise, regular monitoring itself using a glucometer would be of much help in understanding the variations of blood sugar and also in assessing the progress of nutritional and lifestyle interventions(Wukich et al., 2024). Target blood sugar levels are usually defined by healthcare providers. Insulin therapy may be started to attain glycaemic control if dietary and lifestyle changes are made but blood sugar levels stay high. Insulin is usually given via syringes or pens and is thought to be safe for the mother and the fetus during pregnancy. To monitor the health of both the mother and the foetus, evaluate blood sugar control, and modify treatment plans as necessary, regular prenatal checkups with healthcare providers are crucial (Jacobs et al., 2024). In situations when the fatal danger is substantial, further monitoring may be advised. Blood sugar levels in most women with GDM get back to normal after delivery. They are still standing at a significant risk of developing mature-onset diabetes, T2D, in their later life. It would therefore be important to provide appropriate postpartum follow-up care, which entails lifestyle counselling and glucose tolerance testing, based on this ground alone for the prevention or delay of the onset of development of diabetes.

In addition to these main types, there are also other forms of diabetes, such as:

a) Monogenic Diabetes Syndromes

b) Secondary Diabetes

1.2.4. Monogenic Diabetes

One single gene mutation causes a collection of uncommon types of diabetes known as monogenic diabetes. Unlike other types, it results in complex interactions between genetic and environmental factors. These genetic mutations disrupt normal insulin production or function, leading to impaired glucose regulation and diabetes (G R et al., 2023).

Types of Monogenic Diabetes: There are several subtypes of monogenic diabetes, each associated with specific genetic mutations and distinct clinical features:

Maturity-Onset Diabetes of the Young (MODY): Diabetes runs in the family and the ailment usually appears before the age of 25. It is a kind of diabetes that is autosomal dominant and is characterized by modest hyperglycemia and sustained insulin secretion. Most cases of MODY are caused by mutations in several genes, such as HNF1A, HNF4A, and GCK (Tosur & Philipson, 2022).

Neonatal DM (NDM): NDM presents in the first six months of life and is characterized by persistent hyperglycaemia requiring insulin treatment. It can be transient or permanent, depending on the underlying genetic cause. NDM is frequently caused by mutations in genes that encode parts of the pancreatic beta-cell ATP-sensitive potassium channel, such as ABCC8 and KCNJ11 (Gowthami et al., 2023)

Transient Neonatal DM (TNDM): It is an uncommon kind of diabetes that usually manifests in the newborn stage but goes away on its own in the first few months or years of life.It is often associated with abnormalities in chromosome 624 imprinting (Moustaki et al., 2023).

1. **Mitochondrial Diabetes:** Mitochondrial diabetes results from mutations in mitochondrial DNA (mtDNA) and is often associated with mitochondrial disorders affecting multiple organ systems. It is characterized by early-onset diabetes, sensorineural deafness, and other features of mitochondrial dysfunction (Khanam et al., 2023).

2. **Other Rare Forms:** Additionally, there are other rare forms of monogenic diabetes caused by mutations in genes such as INS (insulin gene), FOXP3 (forehead box P3), and GLIS3 (GLI-similar 3) (Redenz et al., 2023).

3. Diagnosing monogenic diabetes requires a high index of suspicion and genetic testing to identify specific mutations associated with the condition. Genetic testing can help differentiate monogenic diabetes from more common forms of diabetes and guide personalized treatment strategies. Management of monogenic diabetes often involves tailored approaches based on the underlying genetic defect. For example, individuals with MODY may respond well to sulfonylurea medications rather than insulin therapy. Early diagnosis and appropriate management of monogenic diabetes are essential for achieving optimal glycaemic control, preventing complications, and providing genetic counselling to affected individuals and their families.

1.2.5. Secondary Diabetes

Secondary DM occurs as a consequence of another underlying disease or from outside source. In contrast to T1 and T2D, the basic fundamental classification of the disease, secondary diabetes is caused by particular circumstances or reasons. Some medications, such as corticosteroids, can prevent the system from either producing or using insulin, thereby elevating blood sugar levels; this can be one of the common causes of secondary diabetes. It may also be caused by other medications; for instance, anti-rejection medications given to organ transplant recipients. Attention in this regard may be paid to the influence of hormonal defects, including Cushing's syndrome or acromegaly, on diabetes induction through the disturbance of glucose metabolism or the formation of insulin resistance. (Amsah et al., 2023).

Secondary diabetes can also be brought on by illnesses like hemochromatosis, which causes the body to accumulate too much iron, or diabetes linked to cystic fibrosis, which affects those who have the disease. Whenever feasible, treating the underlying ethology or disease is part of managing secondary diabetes. This could entail controlling the underlying illness, resolving hormonal abnormalities, or changing prescriptions. To avoid problems and enhance general health, controlling blood sugar levels with medication, insulin therapy, and lifestyle changes is also crucial in the management of secondary diabetes (S. K. Sharma et al., 2023).

1.3. NEED FOR DM RISK ASSESSMENT

One of the important health problems of the twenty-first century is diabetes, exerting a significant toll on individuals, healthcare systems, and societies worldwide. The urgency to address DM stems from its staggering prevalence, its profound impact on morbidity and mortality, and its substantial economic burden. Risk assessment in DM emerges as a crucial tool in tackling this epidemic, serving as a proactive strategy for early detection, prevention, and management of the disease.

Epidemiological Landscape: Globally, 463M persons between 20 and 79 years old are expected to have diabetes in 2019, and estimates suggest that number will increase to 700 million by 2045. Numerous reasons, such as population aging, urbanization, sedentary lifestyles, and poor eating habits, are contributing to this exponential growth. Additionally, there are significant regional variations in the prevalence of diabetes, with low- and middle-income nations experiencing the greatest impact. Given these patterns, developing efficient risk assessment techniques is essential to halting the rise in diabetes-related problems and reducing the strain on healthcare systems.

Impact on Health Outcomes: Diabetes exerts a profound impact on health outcomes, contributing to a myriad of acute and chronic complications that compromise quality of life and increase mortality risk. Uncontrolled diabetes can lead to a cascade of complications, including cardiovascular disease, stroke, kidney failure, blindness, neuropathy, and lower limb amputations. Moreover, diabetes doubles the risk of death compared to individuals without the disease, making it a leading cause of premature mortality globally. Early detection and intervention through risk assessment offer a window of opportunity to mitigate these adverse outcomes, enabling timely implementation of preventive measures and effective management strategies.

Economic Burden: Besides incurring a human cost, there are also significant financial impacts on people, health systems, and economies from diabetes. Health resources and budgets are extensively overburdened by diabetes at an astronomical level of direct expenses of medical bills on treatment and management of diabetes. Financial cost is further burdened by other indirect costs in terms of productivity, disability, absenteeism, and early mortality due to diabetes. Within this context, risk assessment is an economic approach to the prevention or delay of diabetes, thereby containing healthcare expenditures and enhancing economic well-being and productivity.

Preventive Imperative: Assessment of diabetes risk is important because it is central to preventive healthcare. Once people who are at high risk for diabetes are identified, specific treatments may be deployed against obesity, poor diet, low physical exercise, and smoking as modifiable risk factors. This has been evidenced by the fact that changes in lifestyle involving weight-reduction measures, exercise programs for people to improve their physical fitness status, and interventions to facilitate quitting smoking and dietary advice have all helped to reduce diabetes incidence and retard its progression. Pharmacological interventions like giving metformin or other glucose-lowering agents can be considered to test high-risk individuals for delaying or preventing the onset of diabetes and its complications.

Public Health Impact: From a public health perspective, diabetes risk assessment holds the promise of alleviating the societal burden of the disease by reducing healthcare expenditures, improving health outcomes, and enhancing population health Risk assessment helps to promote healthy habits, early diagnosis of metabolic abnormalities, and tailored healthcare delivery by identifying people who are at risk of developing diabetes and putting preventative measures in place. Furthermore, risk assessment informs policy-making efforts aimed at creating supportive environments for healthy living, including initiatives to improve access to nutritious foods, promote physical activity, and create walkable communities.

The imperative for diabetes risk assessment is driven by the urgent need to address the escalating burden of diabetes on individuals, healthcare systems, and societies. Risk assessment serves as a cornerstone of preventive healthcare, offering a proactive approach to detecting individuals at risk of developing diabetes and enabling targeted interventions to mitigate disease progression and its related complications. By prioritizing risk assessment strategies, investing in preventive interventions, and fostering multi-sectoral collaborations, we can collectively work towards stemming the tide of the diabetes epidemic and improving health outcomes for all.

1.4. METHODS FOR DM RISK ASSESSMENT

The Fig 1.1 shows various methods for diagnosing DM.

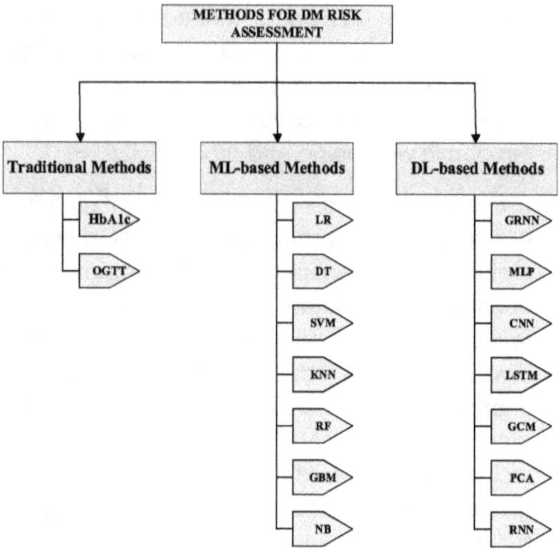

Figure 1.1 Methods for DM risk assessment

1.4.1. Traditional Methods

Conventional tests used in the detection of diabetes include fasting plasma glucose, oral glucose tolerance tests, and hemoglobin A 1 C testing. They are good diagnostic methods but do not give much information on the disease progression and severity of the risk. Recent developments introduce machine learning algorithms like logistic regression, support vector machines and ensemble models and deep learning styles like CNNs, LSTMs, GCNs and attention-based networks. The methods allow automated learning of the features, temporal learning, and integration of multimodal data to enhance the accuracy of diagnosis. The identification of those at risk of getting diabetes has been largely facilitated by traditional methods of DM risk assessment, which depend on recognized clinical criteria, medical history, family history, and lifestyle factors (Yang et al., 2022) . For many years, these techniques have guided preventative measures and offered insightful information about the risk of DM. Clinical markers such as HbA1c values, OGTT results, and fasting blood glucose levels are frequently used in traditional diabetes risk assessment. These biomarkers may not be as accurate in forecasting future risk, despite being crucial for identifying diabetes and evaluating glucose metabolism overall. One measurement, for example, might not account for temporary factors impacting blood sugar or variations in glucose levels over time, potentially misclassifying risk. A fundamental component of traditional risk assessment is obtaining a medical history and a family history of diabetes for an individual (*Diabetes Disease Detection and Classification on Indian Demographic and Health Survey Data Using Machine Learning Methods - ScienceDirect*, n.d.). This method, meanwhile, might miss some risk factors that are not identified by a patient's medical history alone. For instance, complex interactions between several genes and environmental factors may impact genetic predisposition to diabetes in ways that are not entirely explained by family history alone.

Furthermore, risk assessment may be impacted by biases and errors introduced by relying solely on self-reported medical and family history information. Traditional DM risk assessment includes lifestyle factors such as alcohol usage, smoking status, physical activity levels, and food. Even if these variables have a big impact on the development of diabetes, evaluating their effects with standard approaches might not be as precise (Michou et al., 2023). Dietary assessments, for instance, frequently rely on self-reported data, which might contain errors and recall bias. In a similar vein, levels of physical activity might change over time and might not be reliably recorded by self-reporting alone. In traditional DM risk assessment, an individual's risk is measured using a mix of clinical, demographic, and lifestyle factors using scoring systems and risk assessment tools. These instruments offer a standardized method of assessing risk, but they might oversimplify the intricate interactions between risk variables that lead to the development of diabetes. Furthermore, a lot of scoring systems rely on data at the population level, which means they might not take individual variability and distinct risk profiles into sufficient account (Abchir et al., 2023).

Although useful, conventional DM risk assessment techniques have some drawbacks that reduce their precision and efficacy in forecasting future diabetes risk. These drawbacks include the simplicity of risk variables, the use of static measurements, the possibility of errors in self-reported data, and the absence of individualization. To overcome these limitations, risk assessment techniques must become more dynamic and individualized. Advanced data analytics, biomarker profiling, and longitudinal monitoring must all be integrated to increase predicted accuracy and guide focused preventative interventions. Overcoming these obstacles will enable medical professionals to improve diabetes early detection, optimize risk stratification techniques, and finally decrease the burden that people and the healthcare system suffer from diabetes-related issues.

1.4.2. ML Methods

By using large datasets to identify complex correlations between risk variables and outcomes, machine learning techniques have become effective tools for transforming diabetes risk assessment. Unlike traditional methods, which often rely on simplified models and predefined thresholds, ML algorithms can simultaneously analyze multiple variables and construct predictive models that gather the complex interplay of factors contributing to diabetes risk. By considering a wide range of clinical, genetic, environmental, and lifestyle factors, ML models offer a more comprehensive and personalized approach to risk assessment, enabling more accurate predictions and targeted interventions tailored to individual risk profiles. The capacity to improve accuracy by identifying minute correlations and interactions between risk indicators that may not be obvious using traditional approaches is one of the main benefits of ML-based risk assessment (Ali et al., 2023). ML algorithms are highly proficient at identifying complex relationships between risk variables and outcomes by spotting nonlinear and multidimensional patterns in data. With this increased predictive power, physicians can more accurately identify patients who are more likely to experience complications from diabetes or poor health outcomes. Artificial intelligence (AI) models enable more focused and efficient interventions aimed at avoiding or postponing the onset of diabetes and its complications by classifying individuals into distinct risk categories according to their particular profile of risk variables.

Additionally, early detection of prediabetes or early-stage diabetes may be possible with ML-based risk assessment, allowing for prompt intervention to reduce risk and enhance outcomes. ML models can detect minute variations from typical patterns that could point to a higher chance of acquiring diabetes by tracking changes in risk factors over an extended period. Healthcare professionals can intervene early with lifestyle changes, medication, or other interventions targeted at preventing or postponing the progression of diabetes thanks to this proactive approach to risk assessment (Lee et al., 2024). Individuals who are at risk can benefit from improved general health and well-being as well as a decreased burden of diabetes-related complications with early detection and care. Although ML-based risk assessment has many benefits, several obstacles, and restrictions need to be overcome before it can be fully utilized in clinical settings. Ensuring fullness, representativeness, and good quality of data for ML model training is one of the primary concerns. Predictions and risk assessments can be skewed due to biases in the data, such as the overrepresentation of certain risk factors or the underrepresentation of particular demographic groups. Furthermore, interpretability may be hampered by the complexity of some

ML algorithms, such as Deep Learning (DL) models, making it challenging to comprehend the fundamental principles guiding risk predictions. To make sure that ML models extend successfully to new data and populations, overfitting and generalization problems also need to be properly addressed (Alzubaidi et al., 2024). Concerns about privacy and ethics while using sensitive health data are a significant factor in ML-based risk assessment. Maintaining patient and healthcare provider trust and confidence in ML models requires safeguarding patient privacy and making sure data protection laws are followed. To create reliable, understandable, and morally acceptable ML models that can successfully enhance diabetes risk assessment and management in clinical practice, physicians, data scientists, policymakers, and patients must work together. ML-based risk assessment has the potential to transform diabetes care and enhance outcomes for millions of people globally by tackling these obstacles and constraints.

The Logistic Regression (LR) technique is frequently employed in the assessment of DM risk because of its easy-to-understand nature, effectiveness in handling binary classification tasks, and simplicity, but LR may find it difficult to capture intricate, non-linear interactions in high-dimensional feature spaces since it is predicated on the assumption of linear connections between predictor variables. Decision trees (DT) are useful for determining feature relevance in DM prediction because they are simple to use and intuitive. Nevertheless, decision trees may not be as generalizable as more complex algorithms due to their propensity for overfitting, particularly when working with noisy or unbalanced data. Support Vector Machines (SVM) can manage nonlinear interactions using kernel functions, which are very good at finding an optimal decision boundary, mainly in a high-dimensional space. However, SVMs can prove computationally costly even on large datasets, not to mention that good performance is achieved by tuning the hyperparameters. The simplest and most powerful instance-based predictor of DM risk will thus be KNN. Due to the curse of dimensionality, KNN may become overly sensitive to the application of a distance measure as a result, making it less effective in processing high-dimensional data. To increase prediction performance, ensemble approaches incorporate several basic learners, such as Gradient Boosting Machines (GBM) and Random Forest (RF) (Nguyen et al., 2024). Even though ensemble approaches increase robustness and reduce the danger of overfitting, they could be more computationally expensive and difficult to interpret than individual models. NB (Naïve Bayes) is a probabilistic classifier that relies on the independence of predictor variables and is based on the Bayes principle. While NB is computationally efficient and robust to irrelevant features, its strong independence assumptions may limit its predictive accuracy, especially when dealing with correlated variables (Gudiño-Ochoa et al., 2024).

Despite the diverse array of ML algorithms available for DM risk assessment, several challenges persist in their application. Data quality issues, such as missing values, outliers, and class imbalance, can significantly impact model performance and generalization ability. Moreover, the interpretability-accuracy trade-off poses a fundamental dilemma, with more interpretable models often sacrificing predictive power for simplicity. In conclusion, while ML algorithms offer valuable tools for DM risk assessment, their selection should consider the specific characteristics of the dataset, interpretability requirements, computational constraints, and performance objectives. A comprehensive approach involves experimenting with multiple algorithms, tuning hyperparameters, and assessing model performance using appropriate evaluation metrics to derive meaningful insights for clinical decision-making.

1.4.3. DL Methods

Deep learning, or DL, is a kind of machine learning that has garnered a lot of attention recently because of its potential to revolutionize a number of industries, including healthcare. DL algorithms hold the potential to improve predictive accuracy and identify those who are at high risk of developing DM by utilizing complicated data patterns in risk assessment. Although DL has a lot of potential, there are a few disadvantages and difficulties that need to be properly taken into account. Large, high-dimensional datasets are a great source of hierarchical representations for deep learning (DL) techniques, especially deep neural networks (DNNs). In DM risk assessment, DL algorithms can integrate diverse sources of data, including electronic health records, genetic information, biomarker measurements, and lifestyle factors, to uncover hidden patterns and relationships that may not be apparent through traditional methods. Moreover, DL models have the potential to adapt and evolve, continuously improving their predictive performance as new data becomes available. Healthcare professionals may create more precise, individualized risk assessment models by utilizing DL, which enables early diagnosis and focused therapies for people at risk of diabetes (Chuter et al., 2024).

One of the key strengths of DL in DM risk assessment is its ability to integrate multiple data modalities, including structured and unstructured data, to capture the complexity of the disease. DL algorithms can analyze electronic health records, medical imaging data, genetic sequences, and textual information from clinical notes to extract meaningful features and patterns relevant to diabetes risk. This holistic approach enables a comprehensive assessment of individual risk profiles, taking into account genetic predisposition, clinical biomarkers, lifestyle factors, and environmental exposures. By automating the feature extraction process, DL algorithms reduce the requirement for human feature engineering and may even reveal previously undiscovered risk indicators. DL models may uncover intricate interactions and nonlinear correlations between variables by directly learning hierarchical representations from raw data. This allows the models to provide light on the underlying processes and pathways of disease. Furthermore, DL algorithms' capacity to accommodate diverse data sources and deal with noisy or missing data improves their robustness and generalizability in practical contexts (Vivek Khanna et al., 2024).

GRNN is known for its fast-training speed and simple architecture. It may suffer from overfitting, especially with noisy or sparse datasets. Additionally, its performance heavily relies on hyperparameter tuning, and it may struggle with high-dimensional data. Multiple layer perceptions (MLPs) are adaptable neural networks that can figure out intricate mapping between input and output information. They are appropriate for jobs involving both regression and classification and can handle a variety of data formats. Computing-intensive MLP training is sometimes necessary, particularly for large datasets and intricate structures. They are also prone to overfitting, and selecting the optimal architecture and hyperparameters can be challenging. RBF networks excel in capturing nonlinear relationships in data by using radial basis functions to model input-output mappings. They are particularly effective for function approximation tasks and can adapt to complex data distributions. RBF networks may require careful tuning of parameters, such as the number and locations of radial basis functions, to achieve optimal performance(Cuevas et al., 2024). They can also be sensitive to outliers and noisy data. CNN-LSTM architectures combine the strengths of CNNs in feature extraction from sequential data and LSTM networks in capturing temporal dependencies. They are well-suited for analyzing time-series data, such as glucose monitoring data, in DM risk assessment. Training CNN-LSTM models may require significant computational resources and expertise in architecture design and hyperparameter tuning. They may also be susceptible to overfitting, especially with limited training data.

CGM provides continuous real-time glucose measurements, offering valuable insights into glycemic variability and trends over time. CGM data can be integrated with ML models to improve DM risk assessment and personalized management. CGM data may be noisy and subject to artifacts, leading to inaccuracies in risk prediction. Moreover, CGM devices can be costly and may not be accessible to all individuals, limiting their widespread adoption in clinical practice. PCA is a dimensionality reduction technique that can uncover latent structures in high-dimensional data. It can help identify relevant features and reduce multicollinearity, leading to more efficient and interpretable models(Leiherer et al., 2024). PCA assumes linear relationships between variables and may not capture complex nonlinear interactions. It also discards information from the original data, potentially losing valuable insights for risk assessment. RNNs are well-suited for consecutive data analysis, It makes them perfect for DM risk assessment time-series data modeling. They can capture temporal dependencies and long-range dependencies in sequential data. RNNs may be impacted by the vanishing gradient problem, which could make it more challenging for them to recognize long-term dependencies.RNN training can also be computationally costly, particularly for deep structures and big datasets. To sum up, every DL method has its benefits and limitations when it comes to DM risk assessment. To choose the best strategy based on the features of the data and the particular needs of the task, one must be aware of the advantages and disadvantages of these approaches (R & R, 2021). Additionally, creating precise and trustworthy risk assessment models for diabetes treatment requires tackling problems like overfitting, computational complexity, and data quality concerns. Existing management interventions entail lifestyle change, pharmacotherapy, insulin therapy, and regular monitoring. Measures like eating habits, exercise, and early detection are very crucial in postponing the occurrence of diseases and their progression. Nevertheless, a sound remediation highly relies on a timely and correct risk prediction and severity evaluation.

Personalized medicine, digital therapeutics, AI-assisted clinical decision systems, and remote patient monitoring are some of the emerging approaches. The combination of clinical parameters and biomedical signals and imaging data will provide a greater insight into the disease and personalized treatment planning. These strategies provide emphasis on the increased contribution of intelligent computational models to diabetes management.

Constraints and Downsides of the Current Approaches.

Current models of diagnostics are usually based on fixed and single modality data and are not robust, interpretable, and generalizable. Most ML and DL models are overfitted, lack temporal sensitivity, weak multimodal integration, and have poor clinical explainability. Complication detection methods that involve images only (e.g. diabetic retinopathy screening) are often not inaccurate on early or ambiguous cases, limiting clinical accuracy.

Research Gap

The research gap is critical in the creation of coherent, explicable and multimodal detection models that can simultaneously detect diabetes, predict severity and assess the risk of complication. The existing literature does not often combine optimal feature selection, spatio-temporal modelling, and multimodal fusion through the cross-attention approach into a single coherent framework. Also, little attention has been laid on clinical interpretability and real-world applicability.

Need for the Study

This has been necessitated by the increasing burden of diabetes in the world and nations coupled with the drawbacks of the current diagnostic methods, which has seen the need of an intelligent, scalable, and clinically aligned diagnostic system. This paper attempts to solve these issues by offering a hybrid deep learning model that combines optimization-based feature selection, spatio-temporal learning, and multimodal data fusion. The suggested solution aims at enhancing the predictive accuracy, increasing the interpretability, and aiding the early, individualized, and dependable clinical decision-making in the management of diabetes.

1.5. ORGANIZATION OF THE THESIS

The organization of the thesis is shown in Figure 1.2. This thesis consists of eight chapters introduction, literature review, proposed LR, SVM with Bayesian optimization in Chapter 3, proposed method LSTM based advanced DNN in Chapter 4, proposed method Bi-LSTM based CNN with BESOA method in Chapter 5, proposed method DL and ML assisted method in chapter 6, Results and findings in chapter 7, conclusion and future work in Chapter 8.

The detailed description of each chapter is explained below:

Chapter 1 provides an introduction to DM risk assessment, types, methods, and the need for early risk assessment.

Chapter 2 presents a narrative literature review covering the medical background of Diabetes Mellitus, its clinical classifications, the importance of early risk assessment, and an overview of existing traditional, machine learning, and deep learning methodologies used for diabetes prediction. It highlights how diagnostic practices have evolved from conventional clinical assessments to modern computational approaches capable of capturing complex risk patterns. The chapter also synthesizes the strengths and limitations reported in prior studies to establish a clear understanding of current research progress. Together, these insights help situate the present work within the broader scholarly landscape and justify the need for advanced multimodal prediction strategies explored in subsequent chapters.

. Chapter 3 includes ML-based techniques such as LR and SVM their working algorithm with optimization in DM Risk assessment.

Chapter 4 consists of the advanced DNN with LSTM in DM risk assessment. Also, the architecture and working principle with block diagrams are presented in this chapter.

Chapter 5 is composed of the feature selection model and multiple pre-processing phases for choosing the pertinent data, Bi-LSTM-CNN with attention based on DL for the prediction and categorization of diabetes.

Chapter 6 is comprised of a DL and ML approach based on optimization for automated DM risk prediction. GCN and CA-Bi-GRU to extract spatial and temporal data with ELM for classification. Chapter 7 includes the result and analysis of the entire chapters 3, 4, 5, and 6 respectively and chapter 8 presents a brief conclusion for the entire thesis.

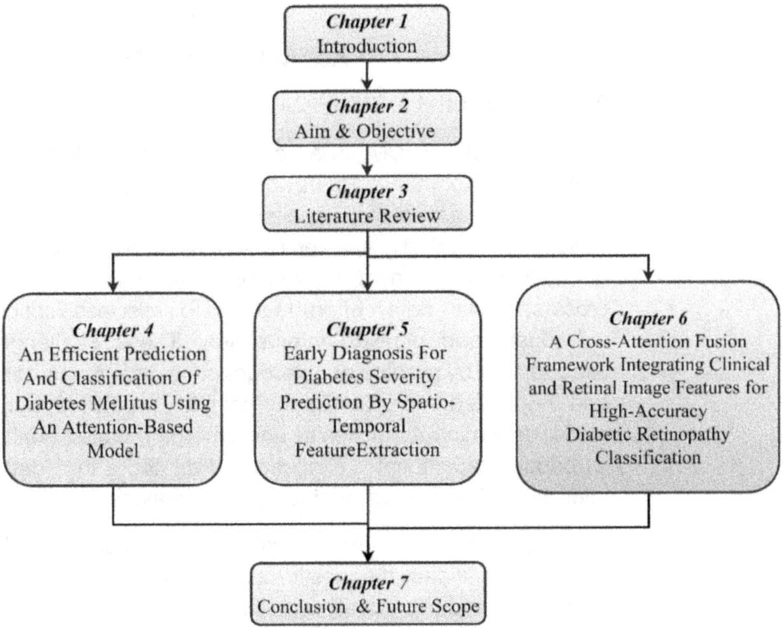

Figure 1.2 Organization of the Thesis

CHAPTER 2

AIM AND OBJECTIVE

2.1. PROBLEM IDENTIFICATION

Diabetes Mellitus (DM) is a complex metabolic disorder influenced by genetic, environmental, behavioural, and physiological factors, making accurate risk assessment challenging due to its nonlinear progression, population variability, and temporal dynamics. Conventional diagnostic and risk prediction methods rely on limited clinical variables and static, cross-sectional data, often leading to misclassification of high-risk individuals and delayed intervention. These challenges are further exacerbated by missing or heterogeneous data, measurement variability, and the limited interpretability of complex predictive models. Moreover, social determinants of health and emerging digital health technologies introduce additional challenges related to data integration, interoperability, and actionable decision-making.

Diabetic retinopathy (DR), a major microvascular complication of DM, presents additional diagnostic challenges. Most existing DR detection models depend exclusively on retinal fundus images, which restricts their ability to identify subtle or early-stage pathological changes that are not visually prominent (Nadeem et al., 2022) ,(Das et al., 2022). Such image-only approaches also demonstrate poor generalization across datasets due to variations in imaging devices, acquisition conditions, and patient demographics(Men et al., 2023), Although multimodal strategies incorporating multiple imaging modalities have been proposed, they often rely on simple or late fusion mechanisms, resulting in weak cross-modal interaction and limited performance gains. Furthermore, the lack of robust interpretability in existing DR models limits their clinical reliability, as predictions are rarely supported by clinician-verifiable, lesion-focused explanations(Y. Li et al., 2023) (Hou et al., 2023). Collectively, these limitations highlight the need for advanced, explainable, and integrative diagnostic frameworks capable of capturing disease complexity and supporting timely, personalized intervention .

2.2. MOTIVATION

The rising global prevalence of diabetes, along with its severe health, economic, and social consequences, highlights the critical need for improved risk prediction tools. Traditional diagnostic approaches often detect diabetes only after complications arise, indicating gaps in early screening and proactive intervention. This motivates the exploration of intelligent, data-driven models capable of capturing hidden patterns across clinical, behavioural, demographic, and temporal variables.

Advanced machine learning and deep learning methods, especially those integrating attention mechanisms and spatio-temporal feature extraction—offer the potential to identify subtle risk indicators long before the onset of symptoms. By enhancing predictive accuracy and interpretability, these models can support healthcare practitioners in making informed decisions and empower patients to adopt preventive lifestyle changes. The motivation of this study is to contribute to the development of efficient, personalized, and reliable DM risk prediction frameworks that can reduce disease burden and improve long-term health outcomes.

2.2.1. Aim

To develop an advanced hybrid machine learning and deep learning framework that integrates spatio-temporal analysis and attention mechanisms to enhance the early prediction and classification of diabetes mellitus risk.

2.2.2. Objectives

- To develop an Attention-based BiLSTM–CNN framework that jointly learns spatial representations from retinal images and temporal patterns from clinical data for early diabetes and DR risk prediction.
- To integrate IBESOA-based optimal feature selection for identifying the most relevant clinical and biomarker features, enabling selective attention to informative inputs while suppressing redundant or noisy attributes.
- To implement weighted multimodal fusion of fundus images, OCT scans, biomarkers, and clinical features to enhance predictive accuracy and robustness across heterogeneous data sources.
- To reduce model complexity and improve stability across validation folds by optimizing feature subsets, ensuring consistent performance suitable for real-world clinical deployment.
- To design a GCN–CA-BiGRU architecture that models relational dependencies among clinical variables using graph convolution while capturing temporal disease progression through correlation-aware BiGRU.
- To enhance diabetes severity prediction by learning both inter-variable relationships and longitudinal symptom evolution, overcoming the limitations of conventional GRU- or LSTM-based models.
- To incorporate attention mechanisms within the BiGRU to emphasize clinically significant temporal features and improve classification robustness.

- To validate the effectiveness of the proposed framework through comparative evaluation and ablation analysis, demonstrating improved performance over baseline temporal models.
- To construct a cross-attention-based multimodal fusion framework in which clinical features act as queries and retinal image embeddings serve as keys and values, enabling clinically guided retinal feature weighting.
- To improve discrimination of borderline and early-stage DR severity classes by enhancing cross-modal interaction between clinical indicators and retinal evidence.
- To achieve robust and accurate DR severity classification by jointly learning from fundus images, OCT scans, biomarkers, and clinical data.
- To assess model generalization and clinical applicability using confusion-matrix-based metrics and external dataset evaluation.

2.2.3. SIGNIFICANCE OF THE STUDY

This study is significant because it addresses the limitations of conventional diabetes risk assessment tools by introducing a comprehensive hybrid approach that integrates machine learning, deep learning, attention mechanisms, and optimization algorithms. The proposed framework is capable of analysing multidimensional, longitudinal data and identifying complex patterns that traditional models cannot detect.

Enhanced early and severity-aware diagnosis:

The proposed optimized and multimodal frameworks improve early diabetes and diabetic retinopathy severity prediction by jointly modelling clinical, temporal, and retinal information, enabling timely intervention and better disease management.

Robust and interpretable multimodal learning:

By integrating IBESOA-based feature optimization, graph-based relational modelling, and cross-attention mechanisms, the study enhances model robustness, reduces redundancy, and enables clinically guided feature weighting for more reliable decision support.

Improved generalization and real-world feasibility:

The modular architectures are designed to ensure stable performance across validation folds and external datasets while maintaining reduced model complexity and efficient inference, supporting deployment in real-time clinical screening systems.

Clinical decision support and outcome improvement:

The proposed AI-driven frameworks assist clinicians in accurately identifying high-risk and borderline cases, improving referral accuracy, guiding treatment strategies, and ultimately reducing the risk of diabetes-related complications.

2.2.4. SCOPE OF THE STUDY

This research focuses on developing a comprehensive and intelligent framework for the early detection, classification, and prediction of diabetes mellitus risk. The scope includes:

- The study focuses on the development and evaluation of deep learning–based frameworks for early diabetes detection, diabetes severity prediction, and diabetic retinopathy severity classification using clinical, temporal, and retinal imaging data.
- The scope includes the design of three modular architectures: an Attention-based BiLSTM–CNN with IBESOA-driven feature optimization, a GCN–CA-BiGRU framework for modeling relational and temporal clinical patterns, and a cross-attention–based multimodal fusion model integrating clinical indicators with retinal image features.
- The analysis is limited to structured clinical variables, biomarkers, fundus images, and OCT scans, with performance evaluated using cross-validation, ablation studies, confusion-matrix-based metrics, and external dataset validation.
- The study emphasizes model robustness, interpretability, and computational feasibility for clinical decision support, while excluding treatment planning, pharmacological recommendations, and long-term patient outcome modelling.

2.2.5. Research Hypothesis

The following hypotheses are formulated to evaluate the effectiveness of the proposed approach for diabetes risk and diabetic retinopathy severity prediction.

H_0 (Null Hypothesis):

The proposed multimodal deep learning framework does not produce a statistically significant improvement in diabetes risk classification and diabetic retinopathy severity prediction when compared with existing conventional machine learning and baseline deep learning models using clinical and retinal data.

H_1 (Alternative Hypothesis):

The proposed multimodal deep learning framework produces a statistically significant improvement in diabetes risk classification and diabetic retinopathy severity prediction by effectively integrating clinical parameters, retinal fundus images, and OCT data through attention-guided spatio-temporal feature learning, when compared with existing conventional and baseline models.

2.2.6. Ethical Issues and Considerations

In this study, we use the JLED dataset (Jothi Laser Eye Hospital Diabetes Dataset) a real-world clinical dataset obtained in Jothi Laser Eye Hospital as part of regular medical check-ups. The dataset contains de-identified demographic, clinical parameters and multimodal ophthalmic data in the form of retinal fundus images and OCT scans.

The data was derived out of a validated repository that had the approval of the Institutional Review Board and institutional ethical clearance. No patient information was identified, and anonymization of patient data was performed before analysis, and thus patient data were collected with the informed consent, and no violations of ethical and privacy standards were noted.

The study is retrospective and computational in nature and has no direct contact with patients, clinical intervention or prospective data collection. The presented deep learning system should not be treated as a substitute to clinical diagnosis or medical judgment and is only supposed to be used as a decision-support system. All the analyses were performed according to the existing academic and ethical research standards, and the results are presented in an open manner.

2.3. An Integrated Attention-Driven Pipeline for Diabetes Risk and DR Severity Assessment

The proposed diagnostic framework in Fig: 2.1 follows a structured, modular pipeline designed to progressively refine information and support accurate diabetes and diabetic retinopathy assessment. Module 1 performs dimensionality reduction and purification of clinical data using an IBESOA-optimized Attention-based BiLSTM–CNN, ensuring that only the most informative clinical and biomarker features are retained for subsequent analysis.

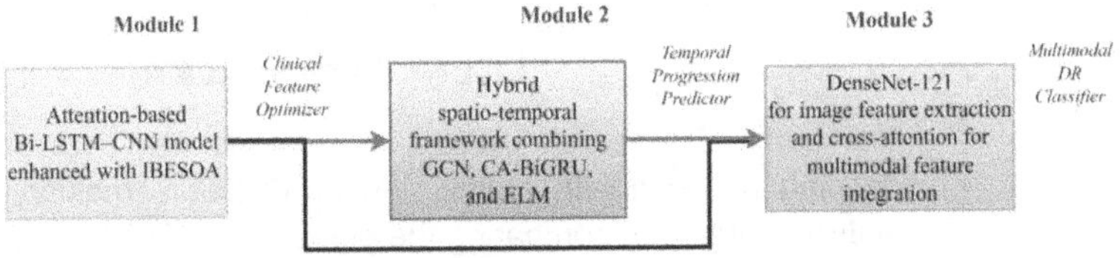

Figure 2.1. Unified Diagnostic Pipeline

The optimized feature representations are then forwarded to Module 2, where a hybrid spatio-temporal framework integrates Graph Convolutional Networks to capture inter-feature dependencies and a Correlation-Aware BiGRU to model temporal risk progression, with an Extreme Learning Machine classifier enabling efficient and stable identification of severe diabetes cases.

Finally, Module 3 combines the severity-aware clinical cues with retinal evidence by extracting fundus image features using DenseNet-121 and applying a cross-attention-based multimodal fusion mechanism. This clinically guided interaction enhances retinal feature weighting and enables accurate diabetic retinopathy stage classification, resulting in a coherent end-to-end diagnostic workflow for clinical decision support

2.4. SUMMARY

This section provides a structured overview of the challenges, motivation, aims, objectives, significance, and scope associated with diabetes mellitus risk prediction. DM risk assessment is hindered by complex etiological factors, data limitations, disparities in healthcare access, and challenges in integrating emerging technologies. Motivated by these gaps, the study proposes a hybrid ML–DL framework incorporating attention mechanisms, spatio-temporal modeling, and advanced optimization techniques. The aim is to achieve accurate, interpretable, and personalized DM risk prediction. The chapter concludes by outlining the research's significance and scope, emphasizing its contribution to modernizing diabetes diagnosis and management.

CHAPTER 3

LITERATURE SURVEY

The body of research related to diabetes risk evaluation is core to defining public health policy, clinical decision, making, and research activities aimed at combating the globally escalating burden of diabetes. First of all, previous studies through their synthesis of evidence, bring to light a broad range of diabetes epidemiology, risk factors, assessment methodologies, and preventive interventions. Such comprehensive reviews allow for the identification of gaps in knowledge, the development of evidence, based guidelines, and the facilitation of efficient risk stratification and personalized care, thus they are instrumental in improving the health of at, risk populations.

DM is a group of metabolic disorders characterized by chronic hyperglycaemia and, ultimately, cardiovascular disease, nephropathy, neuropathy, and diabetic retinopathy as the associated complications. A global surge in the prevalence of diabetes has been recorded, thereby exacerbating the challenges facing healthcare systems, particularly those of low, and middle, income countries such as India. Consequently, the late diagnosis, poor screening facilities, and lack of access to specialized care that characterize the disease have an immense impact on the outcomes of the condition, hence, the necessity of early detection, precise risk stratification, and prompt severity assessment as a means of affording clinical intervention.

Existing diagnostic methods mostly depend on the use of biochemical markers like fasting plasma glucose, oral glucose tolerance tests, and glycated haemoglobin (HbA1c). Although these clinical measures are reliable, they offer only a snapshot of metabolic status and do not depict disease progression, differences between patients, or hidden risk patterns. In the same vein, diabetic retinopathy evaluation by retinal fundus examination and manual grading, even if regarded as the clinical gold standard, is labour, intensive, subjective, and susceptible to inter, observer variability, especially in early disease stages. These shortcomings have led to the emergence of automated and data, driven diagnostic frameworks. The adoption of machine learning and deep learning techniques for intelligent, predictive, and personalized diabetes management is made possible by the advancements in electronic health records, continuous glucose monitoring, and medical imaging. At the same time, diabetes care is progressively focusing on preventive screening, digital health solutions, and decision, support systems, in addition to the conventional glycaemic control strategies. Telemedicine platforms and automated risk assessment tools facilitate accessibility, encourage continuous monitoring, and alleviate healthcare burden, thus, data, driven approaches are positioned as effective complements to traditional diabetes diagnosis and management.

3.1. RECENT RESEARCH IN DM RISK ASSESSMENT USING ML METHODS

(Modak & Jha, 2023) introduced a novel diabetes prediction model that uses several ML methods, such as RF, SVM, NB, and LR. An ensemble learning in addition to these fundamental methods further improves prediction robustness and accuracy. In particular, ensemble techniques were investigated like Bagging, Adaboost, CatBoost, LightGBM, and XGBoost. By merging predictions from several base learners, these methods yield a final prediction that is more accurate and reliable. Ensemble methods often involve multiple models (e.g., RF, GBM) combined together, which increases model complexity. This complexity can make it harder to interpret and debug the model, especially when trying to understand how each model contributes to the final prediction.

(Dharmarathne et al., 2024) presented an ML-based self-explanatory interface for diabetic patient diagnosis. Based on the publicly available diabetes dataset, three classification models were offered: These include XGB, DT, KNN, and Support Vector Classification (SVC). SHAP, an ML interpretation technique, to explain inner workings of these models. While all the models demonstrated respectable accuracy in identifying diabetic patients, the XGB model outperformed the others by a small margin. XGB model using SHAP, offered detailed explanations of logic underlying its predictions at a finer scale. Finally, SHAP's local explanations were combined with the XGB model to create an interface for predicting diabetes in patients. Calculating SHAP values for each prediction can be computationally expensive, especially with large datasets or complex models. This might limit real-time applications or quick iteration cycles during model development.

(Guleria et al., 2024) conducted a thorough analysis of how cloud-based technologies, AI, the IoT, and data science skills come together, introducing data science as a platform for cloud-based service platform to predict diabetes. To do this, a paradigm for data-driven healthcare systems that leverage cloud-based platforms and data science was put forth. For attribution selection, the feature ranking employs MRMR, Relief, and ANOVA, then SHAP. For female patients with diabetes, the Neural Network model is used to make the predictions. Involving third-party DSaaS providers requires careful consideration of data handling practices to comply with regulatory requirements and maintain patient trust.

(Amma N.G., 2024) suggested an attempt to predict diabetes, this study looks at various physical characteristics of the human body. The risk of DM was predicted using an ensemble approach called En-RfRsK, a voting classifier that combines three ML methods: RF, radial SVM , and KNN. RF makes use of output from several different, comparatively uneven models or trees. R-SVM makes use of function whose value diverges with distance from origin. The diabetic data's non-linear decision bounds were learned by KNN. The PIMA dataset was used to conduct the experiments. Deploying ensemble models in healthcare environments requires careful consideration of scalability and integration with existing IT infrastructure. Ensuring that the model can handle large volumes of patient data efficiently and provide predictions promptly is crucial for practical implementation.

(Gowthami et al., 2024) introduced research to evaluate the efficacy of using ML algorithms or early identification of T2D. Utilizing a dataset comprising healthy controls and patients with T2DM diagnosis dataset of patients with T2DM diagnoses and healthy controls, a classification model was built using sophisticated feature selection methods. Using ML algorithms like logistic regression, KNN, DT, RF, and SVM, the model was put through a rigorous training and testing process. The outcomes show that the RF algorithm detects T2DM with an amazing 98% accuracy rate. This astounding precision highlights the enormous promise of ML algorithms in promoting the early identification of T2D. It is underlined how crucial it is to apply these strategies to the therapeutic decision-making procedure. When training machine learning models, having access to representative, high-quality data is essential. In healthcare, obtaining clean and well-labeled datasets that encompass diverse demographics and clinical scenarios can be challenging. Imbalanced datasets (where positive cases of T2DM are rare compared to negative cases) can also skew model performance and lead to biased predictions.

(Xie & Wang, 2020) introduced regression-based models derived from ML and DL, such as Temporal Convolution Networks (TCNs) and Standard LSTM networks, which were included in the ML algorithms. Evaluations had been conducted on a wide range of input feature combinations and regression model ordering, along with use of either direct or recursive technique for multi-step BG level prediction. Blood glucose data from T1D patients can be noisy, irregularly sampled, and prone to missing values or outliers. Ensuring data quality through effective preprocessing (e.g., imputation, normalization) is crucial for accurate model training and evaluation.Time-series data may require special handling for feature engineering to capture relevant temporal patterns and trends.

(El-Sofany et al., 2024) employed ML methods on the PID and private diabetes datasets to run an automated diabetes prediction system. In contrast to other research, this work accurately predicted the dataset's features related to diabetes by utilizing a semi-supervised model in conjunction with significant gradient boosting. The researchers also tackle the problem of imbalanced classes using the SMOTE technique. With the aid of SHAP techniques, explainable AI was utilized to comprehend how the model forecasts the outcome. The study made use of a domain adaptation method to further demonstrate the flexibility of the recommended solution. When private health information is collected and kept on a mobile app, there are major privacy concerns. Ensuring compliance with data protection rules, like GDPR and HIPAA, and putting robust security measures in place to secure sensitive health information are crucial but challenging. Users may be reluctant to share sensitive health data due to privacy concerns, potentially limiting the amount and quality of data available for model training.

(Hennebelle et al., 2024) presented a blockchain-based IoT edge AI system for diabetes risk factor prediction. Based on blockchain technology, the solution can guarantee user privacy and data confidentiality while obtaining a consolidated picture of patient risk factor data from several hospitals. An analysis that compares and contrasts various medical sensors, tools, and techniques to determine and extract the risk factor values inside the system. The researcher used three real-world diabetes datasets to conduct numerical trials and comparative analysis within the system that was provided. Also, employed the most precise RF model along with the two most widely utilized cutting-edge ML techniques, LR and SVM. Handling sensitive health data for diabetes prediction raises significant privacy and security concerns. IoT devices and edge nodes collect real-time health data, which needs to be processed, transferred, and stored securely to avoid breaches or unwanted access. Blockchain technology can offer decentralized and immutable data storage, but ensure data privacy while maintain transparency poses technical and regulatory challenges.

(Chowdhury et al., 2024) aimed at estimating a person's risk of improving diabetes by taking into health and socioeconomic circumstances and minimizing difficulties caused by incomplete data On training data, several data augmentation approaches were applied to lessen the impact of imbalanced data. These strategies included undersampling (Edited Nearest Neighbor, or ENN), oversampling (Synthetic Minority Over Sampling for Nominal Data, or SMOTE-N), and hybrid sampling (SMOTE-Tomek and SMOTE-ENN). The study emphasizes the need of appropriately utilizing data augmentation techniques to prevent data loss and enhance the efficiency of ML algorithms. Furthermore, it gives medical practitioners a thorough ML framework, covering everything from data gathering to ML prediction, enabling them to make decisions that can be justified. The quality of synthetic samples produced can be negatively impacted by noisy and anomalous data points, which were detected by both SMOTE-Tomek and SMOTE-ENN. Model generalization may be impacted by noisy samples that inject biases or erroneous patterns into the minority class.

(Cichosz et al., 2024) created an ML model to forecast the likelihood of new-onset diabetes (NOD) patients developing pancreatic ductal adenocarcinoma. Patients with diabetes associated with a population-based sample of NOD patients older than 50 were included in this investigation, along with 716 instances, and patients with diabetes linked with pancreatic cancer, It is currently described as NOD with a PDAC diagnosis 3 years later.There were 50 in addition to 716 cases. This study included 1:1 randomly matched NOD volunteers and PCRD patients. An RF model was created to distinguish PCRD from Type 2 diabetes using information from Danish national health registries. The characteristics were all the result of feature engineering and contained parameters based on trajectories of conventional biochemical variables together with age and gender. The relative risk ratings and receiver operating characteristic curves were utilized to assess the model's efficacy. Routine biochemical parameters used for prediction, such as blood glucose levels, HbA1c, and lipid profiles, must be consistently measured and accurately recorded. Incomplete or erroneous data can undermine the reliability and predictive power of the models.

(Kumar et al., 2024) introduced a revolutionary ensemble ML-based diabetes prediction system called "iDP." The regular data was collected by the suggested iDP framework using non-intrusive devices, and with the aid of communication protocols, it can be saved in a cloud-oriented storage system. Such a large amount of data makes high-accuracy results prediction possible. Under the category of data pre-processing, three distinct methods have been used: (i) screening, (ii) diagnosis, and (iii) data editing. The model was chosen using the KCV and RFE techniques. This technique necessitates extensive training procedures as well as significant computer resources (such as large-scale distributed computing high-performance GPUs), which can be costly and impractical for deployment in resource-constrained environments.

(Doğru et al., 2023) provided a novel super ensemble learning model that will facilitate DM early diagnosis. Super learner was a cross-validation method that combines predictions from multiple ML algorithms to produce more accurate predictions. Based on a case study, the suggested super learner model was constructed using a meta-learner

SVM and 4 base learners (LR, DT, RF, and gradient boosting). The suggested model's robustness was evaluated using three distinct datasets. Out of five distinct feature selection strategies, chi-square was found to be the best one. GridSearch was also used to create hyper-parameter settings. The chi-square test assumes that features (variables) are independent of each other. In real-world datasets, especially in healthcare and medical domains like DM, features may be correlated. Ignoring correlations can lead to suboptimal feature selection and potentially biased results.

(X. Li et al., 2023) put forth data mining techniques to diagnose a patient with diabetes. The chance of contracting the coronavirus would be reduced if diabetes could be recognized in its early stages and people were made to take care of their health at home. Three steps make up the suggested method: feature selection, classification, and pre-processing. Particle Swarm Optimization (PSO) and Genetic Algorithms are investigated in different configurations using K-means feature selection. Applications for diabetes diagnosis have not before been investigated for these combinations. The diabetes dataset is classified using the KNN method. The k-means algorithm assumes that clusters are spherical and have equal variance. In real-world datasets, especially in medical data like DM, clusters may not necessarily be spherical or of equal size, leading to suboptimal clustering results.

(Dweekat & Lam, 2023) introduced a model to categorize patients with diabetes, this study combines the use of genetic algorithms, multilayer perceptrons, and the model of experiments (DOE, GA, and MLP). In this research, two rounds of factorial design were applied to find the best set of parameters in the GA. In this case, the MLP parameters had been optimized previously by the GA; the MLP enables the fitness evaluation of solution and functions as a simulator within the GA. An optimized MLP was applied to achieve the maximum classification accuracy in diabetic patients, which was demonstrated as the ideal solution arising from DOE–GA–MLP. It turned out that the proposed method outperformed the other eight different algorithms for categorization, considering F1-score, sensitivity, and accuracy. This developed DOE-GA-MLP model can be used by medical practitioners as a very strong prediction tool for the early identification of a person suffering from this disease. Finding the optimal combination of hyperparameters requires extensive tuning and validation, which can be iterative and resource-intensive.

(Mishra et al., 2020) obtained an optimal symptoms dataset, this paper recommended the implementation of a new hybrid attribute optimization approach termed the Enhanced and Adaptive Genetic approach. A probable case of diabetes was predicted using symptom readings from the optimized dataset. Based on the identified symptoms, the EAGA model was further utilized in conjunction with MLP to ascertain if a patient has type 2 diabetes or not. EAGA-MLP, which was the name of the proposed classification method. To evaluate its effectiveness and effects, it was also applied to seven distinct disease datasets. The suggested model's effectiveness was confirmed using some crucial performance indicators. MLPs are prone to issues like gradient vanishing or exploding during training, especially in deep architectures with many layers. This occurs when gradients are too small (vanishing) or excessively big (exploding), leading to slow convergence or unstable training.

(Pethunachiyar, 2020) applied SVM with various kernel functions for DM risk assessment. The accuracy value for the categorization of diabetes was demonstrated by SVM with a linear kernel. The kernel-type parameter's values were taken into account when conducting the investigation. The web link named "Data sets" provides access to the UCI ML Repository, where data sets were sourced from. Selecting the data from the UCI repository and fixing issues such as missing values, inconsistent data, and incorrect information in the data set constitutes the first stage . Training and testing data were kept separate in databases that are saved in text and Excel formats. 30% and 70% of the data, respectively, are used for testing and training. SVMs with linear kernel functions can become computationally expensive and slow to train, particularly when dealing with large-scale datasets or datasets with a high number of features.

(Howsalya Devi et al., 2020)` diagnosed the DM using an integrated method that combines the Sequential Minimal Optimization classifier with the Farthest First (FF) clustering algorithm. The data was divided into some clusters using the FF clustering algorithm. Seventy-eight samples from diabetic patients were obtained from the Pima Indians Dataset and used in the diabetes diagnosis. According to experimental results, the integrated approach that was suggested was able to predict DM with a classification accuracy of 99.4%. The smaller dataset size resulted in a significant reduction in processing time. The clustering output is fed into the SVM classifier as input. It accurately divides patients into those with diabetes and those without, based on test results. SMO requires tuning of parameters like the kernel parameters and the regularization parameter CC (if using a non-linear kernel). Selecting optimal values for these parameters can significantly impact SVM performance and may require extensive experimentation.

(Prabha et al., 2021) recommended a non-invasive method for simple DM detection that is based on wristband photoplethysmography (PPG) signal and basic physiological parameters (PhyP). A dataset comprising

217 individuals with normal conditions, prediabetes, and diabetes was utilised to build the methodology. The Mel frequency cepstral coefficients (MFCC), extracted from 5s PPG signal segments and the PhyP, are used in machine learning approaches. The RF, KNN, SVM, and XGB classifiers were used for classification. To reduce the quantity of input data, a hybrid feature selection method (Hybrid FS) was also proposed. Implementing a hybrid feature selection approach typically involves integrating multiple techniques to identify most relevant features for the XGBoost classifier. The complexity of combining these methods and selecting optimal feature subsets can increase the implementation time and computational resources required for model development and deployment.

(Arora et al., 2022) constructed a model to forecast patient's likelihood of acquiring diabetes with the best level of accuracy possible. Novel architecture utilizing SVM and the K-means clustering technique was introduced for the prediction of diabetes patients. After K-means features were retrieved, an SVM classifier was used to classify data. This method was tested using the PIDD, a publicly accessible dataset. 98.7% accuracy was reported on the dataset that was used. For this dataset, the combination method performs better than the conventional SVM-based classification. Additionally, the, recall, F1-score accuracy and precision of the various ML methods for diabetes patient classification were studied in this work. K-means clustering and SVM both can be computationally expensive, particularly with large-scale datasets or high-dimensional feature spaces commonly encountered in medical data.

(Patil et al., 2022) constructed a multi-class predictive model that used ML algorithms to diagnose type 2 diabetes using clinical data that was regularly available. This study used a modified Mayfly-SVM to precisely identify the prediabetic state. Comparability in efficiency testing of suggested new model was made against T2DM prediction models developed over the last five years. An evaluation of the suggested model was conducted using the benchmark. Two additional datasets—the PIMA dataset from the UCI Repository and one from adjacent hospitals. According to the study, modified Mayfly-SVM achieved a maximum test accuracy of 94.5% by outperforming PIMA and metaheuristic optimization algorithms in both local and global searching capacities. The effectiveness of Mayfly-SVM heavily depends on the caliber and suitability of the chosen data snapshots. If snapshots are not chosen appropriately or do not adequately represent the current state of patient health, the SVM models may produce inaccurate or biased predictions.

(Thenappan et al., 2022) developed a novel, very accurate early diabetes prediction algorithm. The improved principal component analysis was investigated in this work. This analysis extracts features from the dataset more effectively. The ML technique known as the modified SVM (MSVM), which was used to identify diabetes early in the disease, has been proposed to obtain the maximum classification accuracy. This study's primary contribution to cloud security was the mining of the patient's illness data. This security rationale led to the use of the honey bee encryption and decryption technique. The suggested method's performance metrics were assessed using a range of metrics, including negative predictive value, specificity, accuracy, sensitivity, and precision. Storing sensitive medical data, such as patient health records and diagnostic information, in the cloud raises concerns about data privacy and confidentiality. Inadequate security measures or breaches in cloud infrastructure could lead to unauthorized access, data theft, or exposure of patient information, compromising patient privacy and violating regulatory requirements.

(Kumari et al., 2021) primary goal was to accurately predict DM by utilizing a group of ML algorithms. The PIDD, which compiles information on people with and without diabetes, has been taken into consideration for experimentation. The ML algorithms—RF, logistic regression, and NB were combined in the suggested ensemble soft voting classifier to provide binary classification. Soft voting classifiers combine predictions from multiple models, making it challenging to interpret how each individual model contributes to the final prediction. Lack of transparency in decision-making may hinder understanding of the underlying factors influencing DM prediction, which is critical for clinical acceptance and trust in predictive models.

(Maulidina et al., 2021) used the PIMA dataset and was classified using the Backward Elimination and SVM technique. Eight characteristics were present in the 268 diabetic and 500 non-diabetic patients. A feature selection technique called "backward elimination" was used to eliminate elements from the linear regression model that weren't relevant. The appropriate features for the model were anticipated using this strategy. Some benefits of this strategy were that it lengthens the training period, reduces complexity, and enhances accuracy and performance. As a result, SVM's performance increased. The research' findings demonstrated that the greatest performance was 85.71% with 90% data training when the feature selection approach (backward elimination) and SVM were combined. Backward elimination sequentially removes features based on their statistical significance or contribution to the model performance. This stepwise elimination process may lead to the exclusion of potentially relevant features that could enhance the SVM's predictive ability. If important features are excluded early in the process, the resulting SVM model may not capture all relevant patterns in the data, potentially reducing its accuracy and reliability.

(Gupta et al., 2021) employed feature selection Extra Tree Classifier (ETC) in conjunction with NB and SVM classification models to increase model's accuracy. Evaluation of the results was done using recall, accuracy, and precision metrics. The model's improved performance was computed using the k-fold cross-validation method. Based on the experiment's results, the SVM model performs better than the NB model. ETC combines the predictions from several decision trees that it constructs. This ensemble approach increases model complexity compared to standalone NB or SVM models. Managing and tuning the ensemble of trees requires additional computational resources and expertise, especially with large datasets and complex feature spaces.

(Choubey et al., 2021) suggested a strategy divided into two phases: in first part, describe the PIDD and Localized Diabetes Dataset; in second, the set will be processed using two different techniques. First, the technique uses Polynomial Kernel, RBF Kernel, Sigmoid Function Kernel, and Linear Kernel SVM algorithms to classify data from the PIDD and the Localized Diabetes Dataset. The same set of classification algorithms used in the first approach are applied in the second strategy, which uses PSO as the feature reduction technique. For the two previously mentioned datasets, PSO Linear Kernel SVM offers the greatest ROC and accuracy.

(X. Wang et al., 2021) aimed to address the problems in medical data, which are characterized by high feature redundancy, high dimensionality, and very often occurring data imbalance. In this paper, different kinds of supervised classifiers have been discussed to classify the sample data from a diabetes survey with imbalanced categories and complexly interrelated components, while adopting SVM-SMOTE and two-dimensionality reduction techniques for features: logistic stepwise regression and LAA Features: logistic stepwise regression and LAASO; SVM-SMOTE two-dimensionality reduction approaches. The outputs from these four different classes of supervised classifiers are analyzed and discussed, each using one of the four data processing methods. In the case of feature selection techniques, both stepwise regression and LASSO will eliminate the number of features, which may make it more interpretable compared to high dimensionality models. However, the process of selecting variables (especially with stepwise regression) can obscure the clinical relevance and reasoning behind feature selection, making it challenging for healthcare professionals to interpret and trust model outputs.

(Rehan et al., 2024) used the SVM algorithm along with LIBS to identify DM in human urine. Thirty-five urine samples from DM patients with medical conditions and thirty-five urine samples from non-diabetic control subjects were obtained for this investigation. Urine samples from normal and diabetic subjects were taken, and their LIBS spectra were recorded by using a LIBS spectrometer equipped with a laser emitting at the fundamental wavelength of 1064 nm. Using principal component analysis and support vector classifier to process the LIBS spectra, important changes at some elemental peaks in intensity between the two groups [diseased and normal] were revealed. LIBS generates spectral data that can be complex and high-dimensional, requiring preprocessing and feature extraction techniques to reduce noise and enhance signal-to-noise ratio. Variability in sample preparation, environmental conditions, and instrument calibration can affect the quality and consistency of LIBS data, impacting SVM model performance.

(Rufo et al., 2021) suggested a proactive diagnosis strategy for diabetes mellitus to improve or enable early diagnosis in low medical expert density countries. The Zewditu Memorial Hospital in Addis Ababa, Ethiopia, also known as ZMHDD, provided the diabetes data used in this study. Minimal GBM: The gradient boosting framework has recently yielded some highly effective research results, which deploys tree-based learning methods; thus, with their reduced computational complexities, it is fit for application in resource-constrained regions like Ethiopia. The outcomes of the experiment demonstrate how useful the produced diabetes dataset was for predicting the presence of DM. LightGBM models, like other gradient boosting methods, can be complex due to their ensemble nature and iterative training process. Interpreting the final model and understanding the contribution of individual features to the prediction, particularly in healthcare settings where interpretability is crucial for clinical acceptance.

(Hao et al., 2022) introduced an approach based on biased RF and fuzzy SVM for extracting reduced rules. Random forests with bias use the KNN method to recognize relevant samples and develop more trees to diagnose diabetes using key data, thus enhancing the trend of the rules created for diabetic patients. To improve interpretability, standards and limitations were also loosened in accordance with the mistake and coverage rates. Experiments conducted with the Diabetes Medical Examination Data gathered by Beijing Hospital (DMED-BH) dataset demonstrate that the suggested method performs exceptionally well with an equal number of rules in the model (MCC = 0.8802). Studies conducted on the PIDD and the China Health and Nutrition Survey have been carried out to testify to how universal this introduced model was. Random Forests and FSVMs are inherently complex models, making the extraction of simple, interpretable rules difficult. RFs consist of multiple decision trees, each with its own set of rules, and aggregating these into comprehensible rules can be non-trivial. FSVMs use fuzzy logic to handle uncertainty, leading to fuzzy rules that are harder to interpret compared to crisp rules.

(Azad et al., 2022) a unique prediction model for the classification of DM using the PIDD dataset, utilizing the Synthetic Minority Oversampling Technique, GA, and DT. The suggested PMSGD prediction model comprises four distinct layers that make up its structure. The initial pre-processing layer is accountable for managing absent values, identifying anomalies, and over-sampling the minority class. Using a genetic algorithm and correlation, the most significant features are chosen for the second layer. The suggested model was trained in the third layer, and its effectiveness was assessed in the fourth layer using measures such as Area_Under_ROC (AUROC), precision, recall (sensitivity), measure, classification accuracy, and classification error. The suggested method shows low accuracy in predicting DM.

(Mustofa et al., 2023) suggested an RF approach to examine and compare the PIMA and Abelvikas datasets. Both datasets exhibit imbalance; however, the Abelvikas dataset exhibits greater imbalance and complexity due to its larger class count. The RF was selected as one of the ML techniques with the best performance on many diabetic datasets. Extremely different outcomes were found for the two datasets based on the test findings. RF typically handles high-dimensional data well, but selecting relevant features from a large pool can be challenging. Ineffective feature selection or inclusion of irrelevant features can lead to overfitting or reduce the model's interpretability.

(Hasan et al., 2025) have developed an automated deep learning-based diagnostic framework that can classify diabetic eye diseases into four categories, i.e. normal, cataract, glaucoma, and retinal disease. The work has gone beyond just the classification to introducing a dedicated preprocessing strategy that can elevate the quality of the fundus image so that the classification can be more accurate. The proposed architecture couples two state-of-the-art convolutional neural networks, VGG16 and XceptionNet, where a transition block is used to fix the problem of the output feature dimensions of the two models not matching. Moreover, one more auxiliary feature retention layer is added to keep the most salient representations and, thus, to combine them effectively with the transition block output.

(Naveen et al., 2025)have identified the issues associated with the manual diagnosis of DR, which can take a long time, be expensive, subjective, and prone to human errors. They thus researched deep learning-based automated CAD systems to eliminate these problems, which have been found to be more efficient and accurate in diagnosis than regular clinical assessments. Recognizing the effectiveness of CNN in fundus image analysis, the team of authors came up with a hybrid model named EffNet-SVM that distinguished the presence of DR and non-DR from the binary class. The network uses EfficientNetV2-Small to generate the features, and a SVM with an RBF kernel is used for final classification. The hybrid method introduced was better than eight benchmark DL models as confirmed by experiments on the APTOS dataset where maximum accuracy of 97.26% was achieved. The performance metrics presented suggest that the EffNet-SVM model can be used for trustworthy automated fundus image analysis in CAD-based DR screening.

(Zedadra et al., 2025) formulated DRdiag, a multimodal framework for the early diagnosis of diabetic retinopathy, which is capable of surpassing the inherent restrictions of a unimodal image-based approach. The model unifies retinal fundus images with disease duration, which is a clinically significant factor that has a direct influence on the onset and progression of retinal lesions. DRdiag marries a DenseNet121-based CNN for fundus image feature extraction with a Graph Neural Network (GNN) to fathom complex relationships patient-level features. This multimodal fusion unshackles a more in-depth characterization of disease features, thus, leading to a higher diagnostic accuracy. The framework was put to test with the datasets APTOS2019 and Messidor-2, showing a strong and stable performance. In fact, DRdiag on Messidor-2 was able to deliver 0.976 accuracy, 0.957 kappa, and 0.961 F1-score, whereas on APTOS2019 it was able to deliver 0.980 accuracy, 0.960 kappa, and 0.963 F1-score along with high recall, precision, and specificity. These findings attest to the effectiveness and dependability of the proposed system for the automated DR screening process.

CNN models detect moderate DR well but miss micro-lesions due to limited global context. ViT models offer strong global attention but overfit small medical datasets. CNN–Transformer hybrids improve localization but still struggle with subtle early-stage DR when relying on images alone. Multimodal models often use shallow late fusion, leading to weak interaction between imaging and clinical data.Most approaches lack lesion-focused interpretability and fail to generalize across datasets due to domain shift. Subtle lesions like microaneurysms remain poorly captured without multi-scale or cross-feature attention. Many studies still lack external validation or statistical significance testing.

Table 3.1 shows the different ML methods used for DM risk assessment.

Table 3.1: Different ML methods used for DM Risk Assessment

Ref	Authors	Method Used	Advantages	Disadvantages
(Modak & Jha, 2023)	Sandip Kumar Singh Modak	Ensemble ML (RF, SVM, NB, LR, Bagging, AdaBoost, CatBoost, LightGBM, XGBoost)	High accuracy and robustness via model combination	High complexity and hard to interpret
(Dharmarathne et al., 2024)	Gangani Dharmarathne	XGB, DT, KNN, SVC + SHAP	SHAP provides detailed interpretability	Computational cost of SHAP for large datasets
(Guleria et al., 2024)	Pratiyush Guleria	Neural Network + MRMR, Relief, ANOVA, SHAP	Scalable cloud-IoT framework	Privacy and compliance challenges
(Amma N.G., 2024)	Bhuvaneswari Amma N.G.	En-RfRsK (RF, R-SVM, KNN)	Learns non-linear patterns	Hard to scale/integrate with hospital IT
(S et al., 2024)	Gowthami S	LR, KNN, DT, RF, SVM	RF gave 98% accuracy for T2DM detection	Clean, diverse medical data hard to obtain
(Xie & Wang, 2020)	Jinyu Xie	Regression using TCN, LSTM	Effective for time-series blood glucose prediction	Needs careful preprocessing of time-series data

(El-Sofany et al., 2024)	Hosam El-Sofany	Semi-supervised + Gradient Boosting + SHAP + SMOTE	Tackles imbalance; explainable predictions	Privacy issues with mobile health data
(Hennebelle et al., 2024)	Alain Hennebelle	Blockchain + IoT Edge AI + RF, LR, SVM	Ensures privacy with decentralized control	Regulatory and technical complexity
(Chowdhury et al., 2024)	Mohammad Mihrab Chowdhury	ENN, SMOTE-N, SMOTE-Tomek, SMOTE-ENN	Tackles class imbalance via augmentation	Risk of noisy synthetic data introducing bias
(Cichosz et al., 2024)	Simon Lebech Cichosz	RF + Feature Engineering	Predicts risk of pancreatic cancer from diabetes	Needs consistent biochemical data
(Kumar et al., 2024)	Ajay Kumar et	Ensemble ML (iDP with KCV and RFE)	High accuracy; non-intrusive data	Requires high computational resources
(Doğru et al., 2023)	Ayse Dogru	Super Learner (SVM meta + LR, DT, RF, GB)	Robust predictions from multiple models	Assumes feature independence in chi-square
(X. Li et al., 2023)	Xiaohua Li	KNN + PSO + GA + K-means	Novel hybrid framework	K-means assumptions not ideal for medical data
(Dweekat & Lam, 2023)	Odai Y. Dweekat	DOE-GA-MLP	GA-optimized MLP for high accuracy	Requires extensive tuning

				and computation
(Mishra et al., 2020)	Sushruta Mishra	EAGA + MLP	Optimized symptoms boost accuracy	MLP prone to vanishing/exploding gradients
(Pethunachiyar, 2020)	G. A. Pethunachiyar	SVM with multiple kernels	Flexible classification	Slow for high-dimensional data
(Howsalya Devi et al., 2020)	R. Delshi Howsalya Devi	SMO + Farthest First Clustering	High accuracy; efficient on small datasets	Needs careful parameter tuning
(Prabha et al., 2021)	Anju Prabha	PPG + MFCC + Hybrid FS + ML classifiers	Non-invasive; strong signal-based features	Hybrid FS increases implementation complexity
(Arora et al., 2022)	Nitin Arora	K-means + SVM	High classification accuracy	Expensive for large/complex medical data
(Patil et al., 2022)	Ratna Patil	Modified Mayfly-SVM	High test accuracy	Depends on quality of patient data snapshots
(Thenappan et al., 2022)	S. Thenappan	Modified PCA + MSVM + Honey Bee encryption	Secured cloud-based prediction	Risk of cloud data

				privacy breach
(Kumari et al., 2021)	Saloni Kumari	Ensemble Soft Voting (RF, LR, NB)	Improves accuracy with model fusion	Lacks interpretability in individual contributions
(Maulidina et al., 2021)	F Maulidina	Backward Elimination + SVM	Enhances model performance and simplicity	May remove medically relevant features
(Gupta et al., 2021)	Smriti Gupta	ETC + NB + SVM + K-fold CV	Improved model accuracy	High complexity and computation
(Choubey et al., 2021)	Dilip Kumar Choubey	SVM (Linear, RBF, Poly) + PSO	Best accuracy/ROC with PSO-enhanced SVM	Long training time
(X. Wang et al., 2021)	Xuchun Wang	SVM-SMOTE + Stepwise Regression + LASSO	Good dimensionality reduction; interpretable features	Stepwise methods may obscure clinical reasoning
(Rehan et al., 2024)	Imran Rehan	LIBS + PCA + SVM	Spectral data reveals diabetic indicators	Sensitive to environmental and calibration noise
(Rufo et al., 2021)	Derara Duba Rufo	LightGBM	Accurate and fast in low-resource regions	Hard to interpret in clinical settings

(Hao et al., 2022)	Jingwei Hao	Biased RF + Fuzzy SVM	Effective and interpretable rule generation	Fuzzy rules hard to interpret; rule extraction complex
(Azad et al., 2022)	Chandrashekhar Azad	SMOTE + GA + DT (PMSGD)	Structured 4-layer approach	Reported low prediction accuracy
(Mustofa et al., 2023)	Fachrul Mustofa	Random Forest on PIMA and Abelvikas datasets	Performs well on high-dimensional data; handles multiple datasets effectively	Feature selection can be challenging; may lead to overfitting or reduced interpretability

3.2. Inferences

ML methods hold promise for improving diabetes detection through advanced data analysis techniques, its implementation in clinical practice requires addressing significant challenges related to interpretability, data quality, generalization, and ethical considerations. Balancing these factors is essential to harnessing full potential of ML while ensuring safe and effective healthcare delivery.

3.3. RECENT RESEARCH IN DM RISK ASSESSMENT USING DL METHODS

(Mohamed Yousuff et al., 2024) introduced a new use of DL algorithms in the domain of diabetes management, interpretation and prediction of CGM data. In this treatment system, complex patterns and trends of glucose fluctuation can be recognized, given the gigantic database of CGM and supplementary measurements of patient characteristics and lifestyle factors. With the use of RNN and other DL architectures, the model learns from time dependencies of the data that allow it to predict future glucose levels with an accuracy of very high values. It is this predictive capability of the DL model that will allow for the delivery of personalized insight by warning patients and healthcare professionals about glucose excursions before they actually occur.

(Rajalakshmi et al., 2024) provided a DLM with an effective feature selection method for IoT-based healthcare DM prediction. It started by collecting real-time IoT data from the PIDD related to the patients. To rectify the imbalance of data in the collected dataset, the synthetic minority oversampling technique was utilized. To enhance classification performance, missing value imputation and data normalization were next applied to the balanced dataset as pre-processing steps. Next, the hybrid approach known as k-means clustering-based sailfish optimization was applied, which selects the most important characteristics from the pre-processed dataset by performing both clustering and optimization. Lastly, for DM prediction, the chosen features were input into a Bi-LSTM that includes aiming and switching.

(Zhu et al., 2024) presented a BG prediction model that was population-specific and makes use of the temporal fusion Transformer's (TFT) ability to modify predictions according to individual demographic information. The trained model was then integrated into a system-on-a-chip, which was a crucial component of inexpensive, low-power wearable gadget. This gadget used edge computing to deliver accurate blood glucose predictions in real time, and it interfaced with CGM devices with ease via Bluetooth. The wearable device's TFT model execution used very little memory and power, allowing it to provide continuous decision support for over 51 days on a single Li-Poly battery charge.

(Biswas et al., 2024) introduced the DFU_XAI framework to evaluate explainable-driven DL models' interpretability. The SHAP, LIME, and Grad-CAM were three state-of-the-art explanation methods that DFU_XAI used to evaluate five DL models and establish a transparent DL technique. Most of the time, The DFU dataset, is able to discriminate between diabetic foot ulcers and healthy feet, as well as precisely locate diabetic foot ulcers on diabetic feet. A heat map displayed the precise location of ulcer that needs to be treated.

(Aslan & Sabanci, 2023) suggested a novel DL-based technique for diabetes early diagnosis. The PIMA dataset used in the study was entirely composed of numerical values, just like many other medical data sets. This makes it difficult to apply widely used CNN models to these kinds of data. Based on feature importance, this work converts numerical data into visuals that can be used in the early detection of diabetes using the robust representation of CNN models. Three different categorization algorithms were then applied to the generated diabetes imaging data. Images of diabetes are fed to CNN models ResNet18 and ResNet50. In the second, the deep features of the ResNet models were fused and classified using SVM was used to classify the final method's selected fusion features.

(Nilashi et al., 2023) Proposed model for predicting the risk of diabetic using DL techniques. Utilizing clustering and predictive learning techniques, the method was built. The approach makes use of an ensemble of DBN classifiers for DM prediction, Kohonen Self-Organizing Maps (SOM) for data clustering, Step-by-step Discriminant STEPDISC for feature selection, and Singular Value Decomposition for missing value predictions. The effectiveness of the suggested approach was contrasted with earlier ML-developed prediction systems.

(Armghan et al., 2023) employed a highly sensitive biosensor in conjunction with a medical DL model to detect diabetes. The invention of this extremely sensitive biosensor represents a major advancement in the detection of diabetes. It helps to enhance diabetes diagnosis accuracy and efficacy, allowing for better diabetes treatment. Additionally, it decreased the cost of diabetes diagnosis, increasing accessibility for those who require it. The diagnosis and treatment of diabetes may be altered by this new platform, which will make the process simpler and more efficient.

(Z. Yu et al., 2023) proposed the DMNet DM network framework to assess the type 2 diabetes risk in the elderly. We suggest using the tandem LSTM to extract long-term temporal data from multiple diabetes risk groups. The tandem approach, in the meantime, can be used to capture the relationship between diabetes risk factor groups. Using a synthetic minority over-sampling methodology with Tomek linkages, we balance the label distribution. The challenge of high-dimensional features was addressed by applying entity embedding to obtain better representations for the features. We tested the performance with a real-world data set named Research on Early Life and Aging Trends and Effects as a measure for the effectiveness of our suggested approach.

(Madan et al., 2022) designed hybrid DL model based on real-time monitoring was developed for T2DM identification and forecasting. The contributions of this research are four-fold. To begin with, a comparison of various DL models is given. The researcher integrated two technique CNN-Bi-LSTM to detect (and predict) Type-2 diabetes based on experimental findings. CNN-Bi-LSTM algorithm surpassed the other cutting-edge algorithms by 1.1%, according to these performance results. It turned out to be more accurate, sensitive, and specific than other DL techniques with results of 98%, 97%, and 98%, respectively. Accordingly, this proposed model will let the doctor see the real-time statistics regarding vital signs and get all the information concerning the patient based on real-time monitoring.

(Mathew & Sathyalakshmi, 2023) introduced an effective detection system with the ability to identify DM was of essence in detecting it at an early stage. In this present research work, an efficient classification system called Exponential Anti Corona Virus Optimization was developed for DM detection using tongue pictures. In this, the images were segmented using UNet-CRF-RNN and was trained using the suggested ExpACVO algorithm. In the implementation, a suggested ExpACVO was trained to DQN, and a DQN Network classifier mode was used to detect DM. The suggested ExpACVO algorithm was just a new formula that combined EWMA and ACVO.

(Chandramouli et al., 2023a) used a diabetes health indicators dataset, which has 180,000 records and 23 variables like blood pressure, BMI, glucose, and pregnancies, which was employed in this suggested model. As part of the pre-processing stage, any missing values in the data should be filled in using the mean or median. Given that the dataset has more records and properties, when converting high-dimensional data to low-dimensional data, feature selection was used to improve prediction accuracy. Enhanced RFE is the method used for feature selection. RFE was used to eliminate features that aren't as crucial. The RFE algorithm was extended with certain improvements to increase its accuracy and performance, which was known as the Enhanced RFE algorithm. The Hybrid Bagging Classifier was applied to the extracted features to improve prediction accuracy. Ultimately, the output predicts whether or not the individual has diabetes. The diabetic app was used to display this forecast. The app was based on some characteristics, including age, blood pressure, glucose level, BMI, and pregnancy.

(Du et al., 2023) proposed the CNN-BiLSTMAttention fusion model, a DM prediction technique that should have aided physicians in diagnosing patients with diabetes by displaying their state. This model was used to ensure a high accuracy of prediction while improving the processing ability of models for diabetes prediction in complex data. First, pre-processing of the data had to be done, managing the missing values and then normalizing the data. The processed data was then fed into the CNN module for feature extraction. Afterward, application of the BiLSTM module was done to extract the temporal information from the sequence of features. Besides, application of the attention technique was applied to dynamically weigh the various outputs of the BiLSTM module. FCL was added to complete classification of diabetes status.

(Rahman et al., 2020) created a unique model of diabetes classification based on Convolutional LSTM, which has not been used before.

Following that, the effectiveness of the model developed for this study was contrasted with three widely used models: CNN, CNN-LSTM, and Traditional LSTM.The Boruta method was applied to retrieve important features from the dataset, which includes age, blood pressure, insulin, glucose, and BMI. These were very important factors that facilitated better classification of diabetes patients. We applied Grid Search to conduct hyperparameter optimization to obtain the ideal parameters for the models being used.

(Athanasiou et al., 2021) created and assessed a customized method for identifying meal disruptions in T1DM patients. The innate capacity of LSTM neural networks to handle sequential input efficiently is utilized in an ensemble learning approach to generate various ensemble model iterations. The models categorize as positive or negative at the start of an ingested meal based on input sequences of 120-minute continuous glucose monitoring (CGM) values. To conduct in silico evaluation, the UVA-PADOVA T1DM simulator is used.

(Naveena & Bharathi, 2023) provided a hybrid DL model for glucose level classification and diabetes prediction. When gathering data for experiments, two benchmark datasets were employed. Initially, the CNN was used to extract deep-chosen features. Moreover, weighted entropy deep features were retrieved; the Modified Escaping Energy-based HHO was used to adjust weight. The modified Fuzzy classifier is used to process these variables and classify the glucose levels into high- and low-level categories.

(Rabby et al., 2021) presented a novel method for blood glucose level prediction utilising a DRNN model based on stacked LSTM that takes sensor error into account. The erroneous CGM data caused by sensor error was adjusted using the Kalman smoothing approach. The OhioT1DM dataset, which comprises data from six distinct patients spanning eight weeks, can obtain an average RMSE of 6.45 and 17.24 mg/dl at PH intervals of 30 and 60 minutes, respectively. Designing and training DRNNs with stacked LSTMs involves optimizing multiple hyperparameters, the number of layers, for example, hidden units per layer, learning rates, and dropout rates. Finding optimal configuration can be time-consuming and may require extensive experimentation and computational resources.

(Chee et al., 2024) applied a hybrid DL model CNN-LSTM, which accelerated data from wearable sensors on the ankles, knees, and hips in order to categorize diabetes. The CNN-LSTM model is compounded by two convolutions and two LSTMs. The CNN-LSTM can extract significant features and identify patterns for classification through merging the two models. The accuracy measurement of CNN-LSTM demonstrated by the model was at 91.25%, which was greater than the state-of-the-art method. This research, therefore, opines that practice can change in the future regarding the establishment of invasive technologies for the screening of diabetes in favor of alternative non-invasive ones. CNN-LSTMs are also prone to overfitting, meaning they tend to have exceptional performance on a training set but generalize poorly on new data.

(Alex et al., 2022) recommended an effective prediction technique for DM categorization using the values of Deep 1D-CNN. It handles imbalanced datasets with missing values. First, it eliminated the missing values using outlier detection. Secondly, SMOTE was used in an attempt to minimize the impact of imbalance on the accuracy of the prediction. Lastly, a DCNN classifier was used in making predictions, and a particular set of indicators were used in evaluating these predictions. Experiments on the Pima Indian diabetes dataset have returned positive results from the UCI Repository at the University of California at Irvine. It can be disclosed in the result that our suggested algorithm, DCNN, worked efficiently and was much better. A principal weakness of DCNNs is usually their requirement for a large quantity of labeled training data. Given the constraints of privacy, heterogeneity of data, and expert annotation, it is usually hard to get large datasets in medical domains.

(Zhu et al., 2020) presented a DL model predicting glucose level up to the future 30 minutes with a Dilated RNN. This DRNN acquires, compared to traditional RNN models, a much broader receptive field with respect to neurons intended for capturing long-term relationships by using dilation. Also applied was a transfer learning technique that utilized data from several subjects. For instance, on the OhioT1DM dataset, RMSE value 20.1 mg/dl DRNN, 18.9 mg/dL NNPG, 22.9 mg/dL; SVR, 21.7 mg/dL; ARX. The proposed method is much better compared to state-of-the-art glucose prediction algorithms, which include SVC regression models, and even CNN. The results show that dilated connections might be an effective way to enhance the performance of glucose. Dilated RNNs have additional complexity in contrast to conventional RNN architectures. More complexity would be added, thus increasing the time required for training and the number of computational resources needed.

(Chaturvedi et al., 2023) recommended an approach that trains the model using preprocessing, PCA-based feature selection, and PCA. The model was trained using DC-BiGRU-CNN in the recommended approach. This achieves its dual-channel CNN + BiGRU target using an attention technique and a multi-granularity CNN. The suggested approach was contrasted with the widely utilized GRU and CNN models. When compared to the two competing models, the recommended approach performs better. The PIMA dataset was used to validate the efficiency of the recommended model. CNNs and BiGRUs are both computationally intensive models, especially when used in combination. Training such a hybrid model requires significant computational resources and time, which can be a limitation for healthcare institutions with limited computing capabilities. Table 3.2 shows the different DL methods used for DM risk assessment.

Table 3.2: Different DL methods used for DM Risk Assessment

Ref.	Authors	Method used	Advantages	Disadvantages
(Mohamed Yousuff et al., 2024)	A.R. Mohamed Yousuff	RNN, DL on CGM data	Learns time dependencies for glucose prediction; personalized alerts	Requires large time-series data and computational resources
(Rajalakshmi et al., 2024)	R. Rajalakshmi	Bi-LSTM + K-means Sailfish Optimization	Robust feature selection and sequential learning; handles imbalanced data	Complex and resource-intensive preprocessing pipeline
(Zhu et al., 2024)	Taiyu Zhu	Temporal Fusion Transformer (TFT) on Wearable Device	Low-power, real-time predictions; memory-efficient	Edge implementation may limit model complexity
(Biswas et al., 2024)	Shuvo Biswas	DFU_XAI using SHAP, LIME, Grad-CAM	High interpretability of DL models; visual ulcer localization	Interpretability methods can be computationally intensive

(Aslan & Sabanci, 2023)	Muhammet Fatih Aslan	CNN (ResNet18, ResNet50) on transformed numeric data	Converts numeric data to images to leverage CNN power	May lose numeric precision in image transformation
(Nilashi et al., 2023)	Mehrbakhsh Nilashi	Ensemble of DBN + SOM + STEPDISC	Strong combination of clustering and DL	Very complex pipeline; difficult to tune and interpret
(Armghan et al., 2023)	Ammar Armghan	Biosensor + Medical DL model	Accurate, cost-effective early diagnosis	Requires biosensor hardware; integration challenges
(Z. Yu et al., 2023)	Ziyue Yu	DMNet (tandem LSTM + entity embedding)	Handles long-term trends; balances data with SMOTE-Tomek	Entity embeddings can be opaque and hard to interpret
(Madan et al., 2023)	Parul Madan	CNN-BiLSTM	Real-time monitoring; high accuracy and sensitivity	BiLSTM requires more resources and careful training
(Mathew et al., 2024)	Jimsha K. Mathew	ExpACVO + UNet-CRF-RNN	Unique tongue-based DM detection; novel optimization	Tongue image-based prediction lacks general validation

(Chandramouli et al., 2023b)	A.Chandramouli	Enhanced RFE + Hybrid Bagging	Effective feature elimination and classification	Requires extensive preprocessing and tuning
(Du et al., 2021)	Xingze Du	CNN-BiLSTM-Attention	Improves interpretability with attention; accurate prediction	Attention mechanism adds computational load
(Rahman et al., 2020))	Motiur Rahman	Convolutional LSTM + Boruta + Grid Search	Good feature selection and hyperparameter tuning	Training time and resources are high
(Athanasiou et al., 2021)	Maria Athanasiou	LSTM ensemble on CGM data (Meal Disruption Detection)	Detects meal patterns in T1DM; good for intervention	Depends on simulator data, not real-world CGM
(Naveena & Bharathi, 2023)	Somasundaram Naveena	CNN + Weighted Entropy + Modified Fuzzy Classifier	Accurate glucose level classification; interpretable	Complex multi-stage model; tuning fuzzy logic is hard
(Rabby et a., 2021)	Md Fazle Rabby	DRNN (stacked LSTM) + Kalman smoothing	Considers sensor errors; low RMSE	High training complexity; dependent on quality CGM
(Chee et al., 2024)	Lit Zhi Chee	CNN-LSTM on wearable sensor data	Non-invasive diagnosis; high accuracy	Risk of overfitting; data noise from wearables

(Alex et al., 2022)	Suja A. Alex	Deep 1D-CNN + SMOTE + Outlier Detection	Handles imbalance and missing values well	Requires large labeled datasets
(Zhu et al., 2023)	Taiyu Zhu	Dilated RNN + Transfer Learning	Captures long-term dependenci es; efficient across subjects	Higher training time and complexity
(Chaturvedi et al., 2023)	Abhay Chaturvedi	DC-BiGRU-CNN with Attention	Dual-channel deep fusion model; high accuracy	Computation ally intensive; hard to deploy in low-resource settings

3.4. Temporal and Multimodal Learning Approaches for Diabetes Severity and Progression Prediction

Attention enhanced convolutional neural networks improve performance for fine, grained disease grading in retinal imaging. A gated attention mechanism network (GAMNet) for myopic traction maculopathy combines temporal and channel attention with a ResNet 34 backbone and gated attention, along with data augmentation and class weighted loss, thus achieving an accuracy of 93.3% and F1 of 90.0% over 26, 000 OCT scans, and thereby outperforming multiple CNN baselines Zhou et al.,(*GAMNet: A Gated Attention Mechanism Network for Grading Myopic Traction Maculopathy in OCT Images | The Visual Computer*, n.d.). In the case of diabetic retinopathy, a lightweight channel and spatial attention network (CSANet) working on OCTA images achieves 97.4% accuracy on the OCTA DR dataset and 85.7% on DRAC 2022. The network solves the problem of confusion between the adjacent DR severities and the issue of small, sparse lesions by explicitly weighting spatial positions and channels (Fei et al., 2024) (Ma et al., 2024a).

As a complement to classification, automated SS OCTA processing facilitates the quantification of choriocapillaris biomarkers: a segmentation and artifact removal pipeline results in accurate CC masks (Dice 0.831) and shows progressively higher flow deficit percentages going from normal eyes through NPDR to PDR, with statistically significant differences between groups, thus confirming the role of choriocapillaris perfusion as an objective DR severity metric (Fu et al., 2025). To predict long, term outcome, an oblique random survival forest trained on 43, 444 patients with gastrointestinal neuroendocrine neoplasms performs better than traditional and deep survival models, thus achieving a C index of 0.86 and strong time, specific discrimination up to 10 years, as well as recognizing age, histology, TNM stage, surgery, and tumor burden as the most important prognostic variables (Liu et al., 2024). GAN based style transfer architectures have been refashioned for facial expression recognition in intelligent elderly care platforms, thereby facilitating robust affect recognition in both controlled and naturalistic conditions Chen et al., (Q. Chen & Sheng, 2024a) . The Temporal and Multimodal Learning Approaches for Diabetes Severity and Progression Prediction in the existing works are summarised in tab.3.3.

Table: 3.3. Temporal and Multimodal Learning Approaches

Ref	**Focus / Task**	**Data & Modality**	**Method / Model**	**Key Outcomes**
(Zhou et al.,)	Grading myopic traction maculopathy (MTM)	26,616 OCT B-scans, 2,499 eyes	GAMNet: ResNet-34 + temporal & channel attention + gated attention; weighted loss, augmentation	Accuracy 93.3%, F1 90.0%, recall 89.7%; outperformed six CNN baselines for multi-class MTM grading
(L.-S. Chen & Cai, 2015))	Detecting diabetes from clinical data with imbalance	1,937 exam records (Taiwan hospital), 23 lab/physiologic variables; several KEEL bio datasets	Neural-network-based resampling (NNR) + SVM classifier; two undersampling strategies	On diabetes data: PA 98.4%, NA 76.5%, best GM and F1 vs random over/undersampling and cost-sensitive SVM; generalized well to other imbalanced bio datasets

(Liu et al.,)	Survival prediction in GI neuroendocrine neoplasms	43,444 SEER patients with GINENs	Oblique Random Survival Forest vs Cox, penalized Cox, boosting, deep survival (DeepHit, DeepSurv, DNNSurv, etc.)	ORSF best: C-index 0.86; AUCs 0.91/0.89/0.87/0.80 at 1/3/5/10 years; key predictors included age, histology, TNM, surgery; chemo/radiotherapy not selected
(Q. Chen & Sheng, 2024b))	Face/expression recognition for smart elderly care	Lab and natural-condition facial expression datasets	Cycle-GAN style-transfer network; multiple generators, each corresponding to an expression	High recognition rates on controlled and natural datasets; method robust enough for use in intelligent elderly-care monitoring
(Fu et al., 2025))	Quantifying choriocapillaris flow in DR	69 subjects (normal, NPDR, PDR); SS-OCTA	Classical image processing with shadow compensation, intensity-gradient based CC segmentation; artifact removal	Dice ≥0.831; positional error ~4 μm; CC flow-deficit% rose from 9.8 (normal) to 12.3 (NPDR) to 15.4 (PDR), all differences significant
(Ma et al., 2024b)	DR grading from OCTA with attention CNN	OCTA-DR and DRAC 2022 datasets	CSANet: lightweight CNN with hybrid channel + spatial attention (HAM)	Accuracy 97.4% (OCTA-DR) and 85.7% (DRAC); improved discrimination of closely related DR severities and better detection of small lesions

3.5. Comparisons Between Existing DR Detection Models

Existing models for diabetic retinopathy (DR) detection have different pros and cons. For instance, CNN-based architectures like ResNet and Inception show good classification performance for the stages of DR that are mild to moderate; however, due to their limited ability to capture global contextual dependencies, they sometimes do not detect micro-lesions. To solve this problem, Vision Transformer (ViT)-based models utilize global self-attention; however, they are generally dependent on large-scale datasets and, on the other hand, when small or imbalanced medical datasets are used, they are likely to be overfitted. Localizing lesions becomes easier with Hybrid CNN-Transformer architectures since they merge local and global feature representations, however, their dependence on the imaging data only for early DR stages, where the pathological cues are very faint, limits the performance. Some of the recent multimodal fusion techniques also use clinical information along with the fundus images; however, most of them use late fusion strategies which result in weak cross-modal interactions and very little improvements in performance. Besides that, as far as interpretability of the model is concerned, it is still a challenge since a lot of existing methods just give you the prediction without providing the clinically meaningful or verifiable attention or explanation maps.

3.5.1. Key Limitations of Existing DR Detection Models:

Most current methods for detecting diabetes and diabetic retinopathy depend heavily on retinal fundus images. This dependence makes it difficult for these methods to find disease manifestations of the early stage that are not visually apparent. Moreover, many models have a bad generalization problem from one dataset to another, which is due to domain shifts that result from differences in imaging devices, acquisition protocols, illumination conditions, and patient populations. While some studies use clinical features, the fusion strategies they deploy are mostly superficial, which leads to weak cross, modal interactions and small performance improvements. Besides that, present techniques have difficulty in recognizing faint pathological patterns, like microaneurysms, that call for the use of strong multi, scale attention and improved feature interaction modelling.

The interpretability of current deep learning frameworks is still quite limited as these models mostly do not offer clinically meaningful, lesion, level explanations that can verify the diagnostic decisions made. In terms of validation, a considerable number of studies are short of stringent experimental confirmation such as cross, validation, evaluation on an external dataset, and analysis of statistical significance, thus, the reliability and clinical trustworthiness of the results reported are very limited. Conventional clinical diagnostic practices have been mostly reactive and static, providing little insight into disease progression, whereas machine learning, based methods that rely on handcrafted features and single, modality data are still unable to model complex nonlinear and temporal relationships.

Deep learning has yielded strong results in image, based diabetic retinopathy detection, but the majority of the studies have failed to effectively incorporate clinical and longitudinal data. On top of that, advanced attention, based and graph, based models are even more data, dependent, less interpretable, and lack robust multimodal fusion strategies. To be specific, the combination of optimized feature selection, spatio, temporal modelling, and interpretable multimodal fusion in a single framework has not been addressed by any existing work. The point here is the early diagnosis and severity stratification, where intervention in time and with accuracy is of utmost importance. Hence, an intelligent, scalable, clinically interpretable framework capable of integrating medical imaging, structured clinical data, and temporal health records for early detection, severity prediction, and personalized diabetes management is undoubtedly required.

3.5.2. **Inferences**

DL methods hold promise for advancing DM detection through sophisticated data analysis techniques, its adoption in clinical practice necessitates addressing significant challenges related to interpretability, data quality, resource requirements, generalization, and ethical considerations. Striking a balance between innovation and practical implementation is essential to harnessing DL's potential while ensuring safe, reliable, and ethical healthcare delivery.

CHAPTER 4

AN EFFICIENT PREDICTION AND CLASSIFICATION OF DIABETES MELLITUS USING AN ATTENTION-BASED MODEL

4.1. Introduction

DM has become one of the most urgent health issues in the world, being a chronic hyperglycaemia caused by the malfunction of insulin secretion, insulin action or both. Recent epidemiological studies, number of individuals affected by diabetes is increasing exponentially, especially in developing nations, where lifestyle changes and genetic predispositions are major contributing factors. Early prediction and accurate diagnosis of diabetes are vital for effective disease management and prevention of severe complications such as cardiovascular disease, neuropathy, nephropathy, and retinopathy. However, conventional diagnostic methods rely heavily on threshold-based biochemical parameters and manual interpretation, which may not effectively capture nonlinear relationships among multiple physiological indicators.

Data-driven approaches using AI and DL have established remarkable success in disease diagnosis and clinical prediction tasks. These models can automatically extract latent features from complex medical data, enabling improved diagnostic accuracy compared to traditional statistical methods. Despite these advancements, the challenge of high-dimensional and redundant clinical data persists. Medical datasets often include overlapping, irrelevant, or noisy attributes that can mislead the model and cause overfitting, thereby limiting clinical reliability. Hence, developing a robust predictive framework that simultaneously handles dimensionality reduction, feature importance weighting, and temporal dependency modeling is of paramount importance.

DL architectures such as CNN,Bi-LSTM networks have been particularly effective in capturing complex data patterns. CNNs excel at extracting spatial and interaction-based features from structured clinical variables, while Bi-LSTMs can model temporal dependencies, reflecting the progression of disease states over time. However, when employed independently, these models often overlook, relative importance of each feature in contributing to the final prediction. To address this, attention mechanisms have been introduced, consenting the model to focus selectively on the most informative attributes such as Glucose, HbA1c, or BMI, which are strongly correlated with diabetic conditions.

Despite the potential of attention-based deep models, existing frameworks rarely integrate optimization-driven feature selection, which is critical in handling large-scale medical datasets. Many deep architectures are trained directly on raw or pre-processed data without an explicit selection of optimal feature subsets. This not only increases computational cost but also introduces noise and redundancy into the learning process. To overcome this limitation, the present work proposes a novel integration of the Improved Bald Eagle Search Optimization Algorithm (IBESOA) with an attention-based Bi-LSTM–CNN architecture. The optimization component ensures that the model learns from the most relevant subset of features, thereby enhancing both predictive accuracy and computational efficiency.

The proposed model, termed IBESOA-Optimized Attention Bi-LSTM–CNN, is designed to balance accuracy and efficiency in diabetes prediction. IBESOA, inspired by the natural hunting strategy of bald eagles, is a powerful metaheuristic algorithm capable of global exploration and local exploitation. By incorporating this optimization stage before deep model training, redundant features are removed, and the feature space is refined to retain only the most discriminative clinical indicators. Subsequently, the hybrid DL model leverages CNN layers to capture spatial feature relationships, Bi-LSTM layers to model temporal dependencies, and an attention mechanism to underscore critical clinical patterns. Attention-based BiLSTM–CNN with IBESOA integrates IBESOA-based feature selection with Attention-based BiLSTM–CNN and weighted multimodal fusion, focusing on key clinical and imaging features to enhance accuracy and robustness beyond existing methods.

In this module, evaluation using a real-world medical dataset is obtained from Jothi Laser Eye Hospital, which includes comprehensive patient information such as Glucose levels, HbA1c, BMI, Insulin levels, Blood Pressure, and other biochemical markers. The experimental evaluation demonstrates that, proposed hybrid model accomplishes superior accuracy, reduced overfitting, and improved interpretability compared to conventional DLM without optimization.

4.1.1. Limitations of Existing Clinical-Feature-Based Models:

Most existing diabetes screening models based on clinical features achieve only moderate predictive performance (84-89% accuracy), which is insufficient for reliable clinical triage. Many prior studies rely on black-box ML classifiers, such as RF and SVM, without providing feature attribution or explainability analyses, thereby limiting clinical trust and transparency. Interpretability investigations reported in the literature reveal weak agreement between model-identified predictors and clinician-recognized risk factors, raising concerns about clinical validity. Another persistent challenge is class imbalance in publicly available clinical datasets, where non-diabetic samples substantially outnumber diabetic cases, leading to reduced sensitivity for high-risk individuals. Furthermore, feature selection and optimization are often neglected, with most studies utilizing all available variables indiscriminately, introducing redundant and noisy attributes that adversely affect model robustness and generalization.

4.2. Proposed Framework

The proposed research presents an optimization-driven hybrid DL framework for the efficient prediction and classification of Diabetes Mellitus (DM) is shown in Fig.4.1. The model integrates the IBESOA with an Attention-based Bi-LSTM–CNN architecture to address challenges associated with high-dimensional, redundant, and heterogeneous clinical datasets. This unified framework ensures enhanced prediction accuracy, reduced computational cost, and improved clinical interpretability.

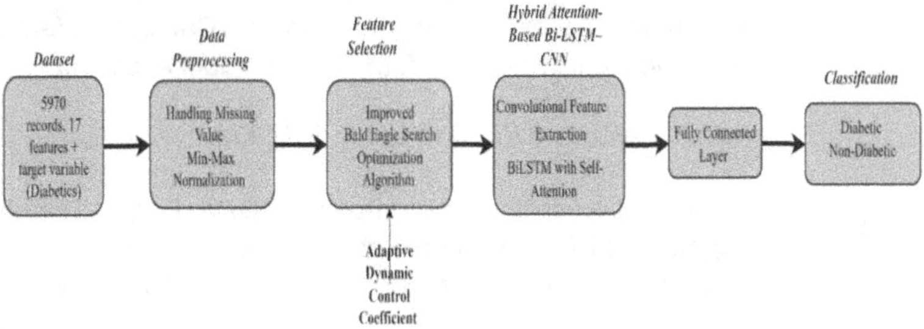

Figure :4.1. Hybrid deep learning framework for the efficient prediction and classification of Diabetes Mellitus

Traditional diabetes prediction methods such as LR, RF and SVM rely on predefined thresholds or shallow learning structures. Although they offer reasonable accuracy for limited datasets, these models fail to capture complex nonlinear interactions among multiple biochemical and physiological indicators, leading to suboptimal generalization performance. Conversely, deep learning models like CNN and LSTM can effectively learn hierarchical feature representations but often suffer from overfitting and high computational cost when trained on unfiltered or redundant feature spaces.

To overcome these drawbacks, the proposed study will create an attention-based BiLSTM CNN model that will be optimized with the help of IBESOA, and the performance targets will be specially defined and measurable. . The objectives are to achieve ≥95% classification accuracy and ≥94% F1-score, while reducing the feature dimensionality by 10–15% through metaheuristic feature selection, without compromising predictive performance. The framework is structured as a three-stage hybrid pipeline comprising data preprocessing, IBESOA-based feature optimization, and deep neural classification to ensure robustness, computational efficiency, and interpretability. Model effectiveness and generalization capability are quantitatively evaluated using k-fold cross-validation and standard performance metrics, enabling objective comparison against baseline and state-of-the-art methods.

4.2.1. Data Preprocessing

The preprocessing stage prepares the clinical dataset for optimization and model training. It involves several essential steps, including data cleaning, normalization, and encoding. Missing or inconsistent values are handled using statistical imputation techniques to maintain data integrity. All numerical attributes are scaled to a uniform range using Min–Max normalization, ensuring that features with higher numeric ranges do not govern the model's learning progression. Categorical features, if any, are transformed into numeric form through label encoding.

4.2.2. Feature Selection using IBESOA

After preprocessing, the Improved Bald Eagle Search Optimization Algorithm (IBESOA) is employed to recognize the most relevant clinical features and eliminate redundant or weakly correlated ones. IBESOA is a metaheuristic optimization method enthused by, hunting behaviour of bald eagles, which alternates between exploration, exploitation, and convergence phases to locate optimal solutions.

In this research, IBESOA is utilized to select the most discriminative clinical attributes such as Glucose, HbA1c, BMI, Age, and Insulin, which have significant clinical relevance to diabetes prediction. By optimizing the feature subset, IBESOA reduces data dimensionality, mitigates overfitting, and enhances computational efficiency. The algorithm ensures an adaptive balance between global exploration (searching for potential feature combinations) and local exploitation (refining the selection toward optimal subsets), resulting in a feature set that maximizes classification performance.

4.2.3. Classification using Attention-based Bi-LSTM–CNN

The optimized features obtained from the IBESOA stage are then passed to the Attention-based Bi-LSTM–CNN for classification. CNN layers extract spatial relationships among the clinical parameters, identifying interactions such as those between Glucose–HbA1c or BMI–Age, which are critical indicators of diabetic risk.

Bi-LSTM layers capture temporal dependencies in forward and backward directions, learning trends or progression patterns across patient health parameters. The attention mechanism further enhances interpretability by assigning higher weights to the most influential clinical attributes (e.g., HbA1c and Glucose), ensuring that the model focuses primarily on critical indicators while suppressing less relevant features. This hybrid integration allows the model to achieve superior feature representation and decision-making capability while maintaining interpretability and robustness.

Workflow of the proposed module depicted in Figure 4.2, outlines major stages of the process.

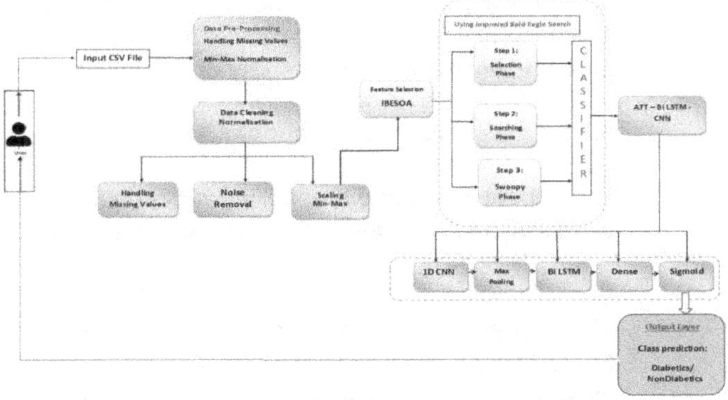

Figure 4.2: *Proposed Workflow of IBESOA Optimized Attention-Based Bi-LSTM–CNN Framework*

4.3. Data Preprocessing

The first stage of the proposed framework involves data preprocessing, which ensures clean consistent, and properly structured clinical dataset, for subsequent optimization and model training. The stage is important in improving data quality, reduction of noise, and promoting effective learning. The data in this study is made up of 5970 clinical records which each have 14 features and a target variable which is the presence or absence of diabetes. The data is organized in tabular format, comprising clinical and physiological parameters such as Glucose, BMI, Insulin, Age, BP, and HbA1c levels.

The preprocessing operations include three main steps: data cleaning, normalization, and scaling, as described below.

4.3.1. Handling Missing Value

In any real-world clinical dataset, missing values (MVs) are common due to incomplete medical records, inaccurate measurements, device malfunctions, or human error during data entry. The dataset used in this study includes several clinical parameters such as Glucose, HbA1c, BMI, Insulin, and Age, where some entries are missing or represented as zero values. Proper handling of missing data is essential to preserve data integrity and enhance the predictive reliability.

Missing data pattern in this dataset follows a MAR mechanism, where absence of certain feature values be contingent on other observed variables. To address this, median imputation was employed, replacing each missing entry with the median of the corresponding attribute. This approach maintains the statistical distribution of the dataset, minimizes bias, and improves model stability during training.

4.3.1.1. Missing at Random (MAR)

In MAR, likelihood of a missing value depends on other observed variables but not on the missing variable itself. It is expressed as:

$$P(Y \mid X, \emptyset) = P(Y_a \mid \emptyset) \tag{4.1}$$

This implies that missingness can be predicted using information from the remaining observed variables. For instance, if the Insulin value is missing, it may be estimated based on correlated features such as Glucose or BMI. Under this condition, statistical or imputation techniques, such as median imputation or regression-based estimation, can be effectively applied to approximate the missing values (Pham et al., 2022).

4.3.2. Min–Max Normalization

To ensure uniform feature scaling and accelerate model convergence, Min–Max normalization is applied to all numeric attributes. This technique transforms each feature value into a normalized range between **0 and 1**, using the formula:

$$x_{norm} = \frac{x - x_{min}}{x_{max} - x_{min}} \tag{4.2}$$

Normalization ensures features with large numerical ranges do not govern those with smaller ranges, thereby improving the model's training stability and convergence (Shantal et al., 2023).

4.3.3. K-Fold Cross-Validation

For reliable model evaluation, K-Fold Cross-Validation was implemented. Dataset was divided into k equal subsets, where each-fold served as the testing set and the remaining $k - 1$folds as the training set in each iteration. This was repeated k times, and the final performance was obtained by averaging results across all folds (Nti & Aning, 2021).

Stratified K-Fold was used to preserve the class distribution between diabetic and non-diabetic samples. Various k values (3, 5, 7, 10, 15, and 20) were tested, and 5-fold CV if the best trade-off between computational cost and prediction reliability for IBESOA-optimized Attention Bi-LSTM–CNN model.

4.3.4. Feature Selection using IBESOA

The IBESOA is employed in this study to identify the most informative clinical features for diabetes prediction. Feature selection is essential for enhancing model accuracy, reducing redundant information, lowering computational overhead, and improving interpretability especially in clinical datasets that commonly contain noisy or irrelevant parameters.

IBESOA extends the standard Bald Eagle Search (BES) algorithm by incorporating an Adaptive Dynamic Control Coefficient (ADCC) to accomplish a better balance among exploration and exploitation during optimization. BES mimics the hunting strategies of bald eagles through three phases: selecting space, searching space, and swooping. IBES enhances these phases by dynamically adjusting the search intensity using the ADCC.

4.3.4.1. Feature Selection Objective

Given a dataset $D = \{(P_i, Q_i)\}_{i=1}^{n}$, where $P_i = [p_{i1}, p_{i2}, \ldots, p_{im}]$ represents m clinical features and y_i denotes the target class (Diabetic/Non-Diabetic), the goal of IBES-based feature selection is to determine an optimal subset of features $S^* \subseteq \{1,2,\ldots,m\}$ that minimizes classification error while maximizing number of informative features.

The optimization problem can be defined as:

$$\min_{S \subseteq F} J(S) = \alpha \cdot \text{Error}(S) + (1 - \alpha) \cdot \frac{|S|}{|F|} \tag{4.3}$$

where: Error(S): classification error of the model trained using selected subset S, $|S|$: number of selected features, $|F|$: total number of features, $\alpha \in [0,1]$: trade-off coefficient controlling balance between accuracy and feature reduction.

Encoding and Fitness Evaluation

Each bald eagle (candidate solution) is represented as binary vector of length m, each bit corresponds a feature:

$$P_i = [p_1, p_2, \ldots, p_m], p_j = \begin{cases} 1, & \text{if feature } j \text{ is selected} \\ 0, & \text{otherwise} \end{cases} \tag{4.4}$$

The fitness function for evaluating each solution is formulated as:

$$f_i = \omega_1 \cdot \big(1 - \text{Accuracy}(P_i)\big) + \omega_2 \cdot \frac{\sum_{j=1}^{m} p_j}{m} \tag{4.5}$$

where:

- $\text{Accuracy}(P_i)$: classification accuracy of Bi-LSTM–CNN using the selected features,
- $\omega_1$and ω_2: weighting factors $(\omega_1 + \omega_2 = 1)$ controlling the balance between accuracy maximization and feature minimization.

This formulation ensures that the IBES algorithm searches for subsets that provide high accuracy with fewer features, avoiding overfitting and improving computational efficiency.

Initialization and Wrapper-Based Optimization

IBESOA initializes a random population of Nindividuals, each of dimension dim, within the defined upper (ub) and lower (lb) bounds:

$$P_i^j = lb + rand \times (ub - lb), i = 1,2, \ldots, N; j = 1,2, \ldots, \text{dim} \tag{4.6}$$

where $rand \in [0,1]$. Each individual's fitness is evaluated using problem-specific objective function. IBESOA and Att-BiLSTM-CNN are integrated through a wrapper-based optimization loop in which IBESOA controls the input space of the neural network. IBESOA first generates a binary mask $s \in \{0,1\}^D$that represents a candidate subset of features. This mask is applied to the original input to create a reduced feature vector $X_s = X \odot s^\top$. The masked input $X_s$is then fed into the Att-BiLSTM-CNN, which is trained to obtain model parameters $w^*(s)$by minimizing the classification loss:

$$w^*(s) = \arg\min_w \mathcal{L}(f_w(X_s), y). \tag{4.7}$$

The validation accuracy of this trained network directly determines IBESOA's fitness function:

$$\text{Fitness}(s) = \lambda\big(1 - \text{Acc}_{val}(f_{w^*(s)})\big) + (1-\lambda)\frac{|S|}{D}. \tag{4.8}$$

where: $\text{Acc}_{val}(f_{w^*(s)})$is the validation accuracy of the Att-BiLSTM–CNN using selected feature subset S, $|S|$: number of selected features, D: total number of available features, and $\boldsymbol{\alpha} \in [0,1]$controls trade-off between classification accuracy and feature reduction (higher αemphasizes accuracy, while lower αfavors compact feature subsets).

IBESOA iteratively updates the mask $s$to maximize the Att-BiLSTM-CNN's validation accuracy, meaning the evolutionary search is guided entirely by the network's performance. The final selected mask is then used as the fixed input configuration for the full training of the Att-BiLSTM-CNN. Thus, IBESOA directly controls which features the neural network receives, while the network's accuracy governs IBESOA's search (S. R. Sharma et al., 2023).

4.3.4.2. Adaptive Dynamic Control Coefficient (ADCC)

To dynamically control the search behaviour, an adaptive coefficient $\eta(t) \in (0,1]$is introduced. It adjusts the exploration–exploitation balance based on the iteration progress and population diversity. To enhance the convergence stability and dynamic balance between exploration and exploitation, an Adaptive Dynamic Control Coefficient $\eta(t)$is introduced. This adaptive factor modifies the movement equations dynamically based on population diversity and iteration progress.

Let t : current iteration, and T_{max} be the maximum number of iterations. The population of IBES is represented as $\{X_i(t)\}_{i=1}^{P}$with fitness values $f_i(t)$.

Defining population fitness variance as:

$$\sigma f(t) = \left(1/_P\right)\sum_i \left(f_i(t) - \bar{f}(t)\right)^2 \tag{4.9}$$

Where $\bar{f}(t) = \frac{1}{P}\sum_{i=1}^{P} f_i(t)$. The normalized iteration progress and fitness variance are computed as:

$$\gamma(t) = \frac{t}{T_{max}} \in [0,1], \hat{\sigma}_f(t) = \frac{\sigma_f(t)}{\sigma_f(0)+\delta} \tag{4.9a}$$

Then, the adaptive control coefficient is defined as:

$$\eta(t) = (1-\gamma(t)^{\kappa}) \cdot \exp\left(-\lambda\hat{\sigma}_f(t)\right) + \epsilon \tag{4.10}$$

where:$\kappa \in [1,3]$controls iteration decay, $\boldsymbol{\lambda} \in [1,10]$regulates sensitivity to population fitness variance, δprevents division by zero, and $\epsilon \in$

(0,0.2]ensures minimum exploration. At early iterations, higher values of $\eta(t)$promote exploration, while lower values at later stages emphasize exploitation, enabling stable convergence and adaptive search behavior.

4.3.4.3. Select Space

In this phase, the bald eagle explores the environment to identify potential regions of interest. The updated position is influenced by both the global best and mean population, modulated by the adaptive control coefficient:

$$P_i^{\text{new}} = P_b + \eta(t) \cdot R_{\text{rand}} \cdot (P_m - P_i) \quad (4.11)$$

where $P_b$is the best solution, $P_m$is the population mean, and $R_{rand} \in (0,1)$is a stochastic factor. The integration of $\eta(t)$ensures that search intensity dynamically adjusts with iteration progress and diversity.

4.3.4.4. Search Space

During the prey-seeking phase, eagles refine their search near the identified promising areas. The improved formulation is:

$$P_i^{\text{new}} = P_i + \eta(t)[x_i(P_i - P_m) + y_i(P_i - P_{i+1})] \quad (4.12)$$

where $x_i, y_i$are derived from spiral flight trajectories:

$$x_i = \frac{x_{ri}}{max(|x_r|)}, y_i = \frac{y_{ri}}{max(|y_r|)}, \quad (4.13)$$

$$x_{ri} = r_i\sin(\theta_i), y_{ri} = r_i\cos(\theta_i) \quad (4.14)$$

$$r_i = \theta_i + R \cdot R_{rand}, \theta_i = a\pi R_{rand} \quad (4.15)$$

The use of $\eta(t)$adaptively tunes the spiral's amplitude, improving convergence speed and avoiding local minima. where $R \in [0.5,2]$and $a \in [5,10]$are random parameters controlling the spiral trajectory. This step increases search efficiency by balancing local and global exploration.

4.3.4.5. Swooping

In the final swooping phase, individuals converge toward the global best solution:

$$P_i^{\text{new}} = R_{\text{rand}} P_b + \eta(t)[x_{1i}(P_i - c_1 P_m) + y_{1i}(P_i - c_2 P_b)] \quad (4.16)$$

where $c_1, c_2 \in [1,2]$control the influence of average and best positions. The inclusion of $\eta(t)$ensures smooth transition from global exploration to local exploitation as iterations progress.

Where P_b= best position found so far, P_m= mean population position, $\eta(t)$= adaptive dynamic control coefficient, $R_{rand} \in (0,1)$= random coefficient ensuring stochastic movement

The coefficients x_{1i} and y_{1i} are defined in polar coordinates as:

$$x_{1i} = \frac{x_{ri}}{max(|x_r|)}, y_{1i} = \frac{y_{ri}}{max(|y_r|)} \quad (4.17)$$

$$x_{ri} = r_i \sinh(\theta_i), y_{ri} = r_i \cosh(\theta_i) \quad (4.18)$$

$$r_i = \theta_i, \theta_i = a\pi R_{rand} \quad (4.19)$$

where $a \in [5,10]$ controls the shape of the swooping trajectory.

The inclusion of $\eta(t)$ ensures adaptive contraction of the swooping radius, allowing stronger convergence during exploitation phases while maintaining adequate diversity when stagnation is detected. where $c_1, c_2 \in [1,2]$ are constants determining the intensity of motion toward the optimal and average positions, respectively.

This phase refines exploitation by ensuring all individuals converge toward the optimal solution. IBESOA refines feature subsets through sequential selection, searching, and swooping phases, where each iteration updates the feature vector by removing weak or redundant attributes and retaining the most predictive clinical indicators. The final optimized subset supports the objective by enhancing performance of Attention-BiLSTM-CNN model through only the most relevant features.

Pseudocode: IBESOA based Feature Selection

Input: Dataset $D = \{X_i, Y_i\}, i = 1,2, \dots n$, number of features m,
population size P, maximum iterations T_{max},
trade-off weights $(\alpha, \omega_1, \omega_2)$

Output: Optimal feature subset S^*

#Initialization
Generate initial population $\{X_i(0)\} i = 1,2 \dots . P$, where each X_i is a binary vector of length m
For each solution $X_i(0)$
Evaluate fitness $f_i(0)$ using:

$$f_i = \omega_1 \cdot (1 - \text{Accuracy}(X_i)) + \omega_2 \cdot \frac{\sum_{j=1}^{m} x_j}{m}$$

Set $P_b = best\ solution$ based on minimum fitness
Compute initial fitness variance $\sigma f(0)$
Main Optimization Loop
For $t = 1\ to\ T_{max}$ do
#Adaptive Control Coefficient
Compute normalized iteration progress:

$$\gamma(t) = t \,/\, Tmax$$

Compute current fitness variance:

$$\sigma f(t) = (1/p)\sum_i (f_i(t) - \bar{f}(t))^2$$

Compute adaptive coefficient:

$$\eta(t) = (1 - \gamma(t)^{\kappa}) \cdot \exp\left(-\lambda\hat{\sigma}_f(t)\right) + \epsilon$$

#Phase 1: Select Space
Compute population mean P_m
For each individual $Pi(t)$

$$P_i^{\text{new}} = P_b + \eta(t) \cdot R_{\text{rand}} \cdot (P_m - P_i)$$

#Phase 2: Search Space
For eachP_i^{new} :
Compute spiral flight parameters:

$$x_{ri} = r_i\sin(\theta_i), y_{ri} = r_i\cos(\theta_i)$$
$$r_i = \theta_i + R \cdot R_{rand}, \theta_i = a\pi R_{rand}$$

Normalize:

$$x_i = \frac{x_{ri}}{max(|x_r|)}, y_i = \frac{y_{ri}}{max(|y_r|)}$$

Update:

$$P_i^{\text{new}} = P_i + \eta(t)[x_i(P_i - P_m) + y_i(P_i - P_{i+1})]$$

#Phase 3: Swooping
For each P_i^{new} :
Compute swooping parameters:

$$x_{1i} = \frac{x_{ri}}{max(|x_r|)}, y_{1i} = \frac{y_{ri}}{max(|y_r|)}$$

$$P_i^{\text{new}} = R_{\text{rand}}\, P_b + \eta(t)[x_{1i}(P_i - c_1P_m) + y_{1i}(P_i - c_2P_b)]$$

Boundary Check & Binarization
Apply sigmoid transfer or thresholding on P_i^{new}
Map P_i^{new} to binary $\{0,1\}$^m (selected/not selected)
#Update Global Best
If $f_i(t) < f(P_b)$ then
$P_b = P_i^{\text{new}}$
End For
Return S^* = indices where $P_b(j) = 1$
End Algorithm

IBESOA demonstrates faster convergence toward an optimal feature subset, particularly in high-dimensional clinical data, where genetic algorithms and particle swarm optimization often exhibit slow or unstable convergence behaviour. The algorithm also preserves feature diversity through adaptive exploration mechanisms, avoiding premature convergence commonly observed in genetic algorithms and early particle clustering in particle swarm optimization. Moreover, features selected using IBESOA yield higher model stability, as evidenced by reduced performance variance across validation folds, whereas GA- and PSO-based feature selection results in greater performance fluctuations due to stochastic mutation and velocity update processes

4.4. Hybrid Attention-Based Bi-LSTM–CNN Model

Optimized features obtained from IBESOA are fed into Attention-based Bi-LSTM–CNN hybrid model for classification. This leverages the strengths of CNN for spatial feature extraction and Bi-LSTM layers seizing temporal dependencies, while an attention mechanism enhances interpretability by emphasizing the most informative features. Although CNN–LSTM–attention frameworks exist, our approach uniquely integrates IBESOA-based optimal feature selection with the Attention-based BiLSTM–CNN, enabling to selectively focus on the most pertinent clinical and imaging features. Furthermore, we employ weighted multimodal fusion of fundus images, OCT scans, biomarkers, and clinical data, collectively improving prediction accuracy, robustness, and generalizability beyond existing methods.

4.4.1. Convolutional Feature Extraction

The CNN module serves as the first feature extraction component of hybrid Attention-based Bi-LSTM–CNN model. Although clinical dataset consisting numerical attributes rather than images, the selected clinical parameters can be structured as a 1D sequence, where the positional arrangement preserves the inherent relationships among medical indicators. Applying 1D convolution enables the model to automatically learn local interaction patterns between adjacent or physiologically related features, which are highly significant in metabolic and endocrinological processes.

Let the optimized feature vector represented as:

$$X = [x_1, x_2, \dots, x_d] \in \mathbb{R}^d \tag{4.20}$$

A 1D convolution operation with Kfilters is applied to this sequence. For the k^{th}filter $W_k$of kernel size f, the convolutional response at position $i$is expressed as:

$$h_k(i) = \sigma\left(\sum_{j=0}^{f-1} W_k(j) \cdot x_{i+j} + b_k\right) \tag{4.21}$$

Where, $h_k(i)$is the activation at position $i$for filter k, $W_k(j)$represents the j^{th}weight of the convolution filter, b_k:corresponding bias term, $\sigma(\cdot)$: ReLU activation function.

This operation slides each filter across the feature sequence, allowing CNN to learn short-range dependent patterns that frequently co-occur in diabetic clinical profiles. For instance, clusters such as *(Glucose → HbA1c)* or *(BMI → Insulin → Blood Pressure)* often exhibit strong medical interdependence, and capturing such localized relationships enhances the discriminative capacity of the classifier.

The resulting convolutional output, or feature map, is represented as:

$$H = [h_1, h_2, \dots, h_K] \in \mathbb{R}^{L \times K} \tag{4.22}$$

where:

- Kdenotes the number of convolution filters,
- $L$is the output sequence length after convolution, determined by the kernel size and padding.

The convergence behavior directly influences the prediction metrics because faster and more stable convergence leads to the selection of an optimal, non-redundant feature subset. Since IBESOA achieves early and stable convergence compared to PSO and GA, the resulting feature subset is more discriminative, which in turn improves the downstream classification metrics. Therefore, IBESOA's convergence advantage directly contributes to its superior predictive performance.

4.4.2. Bidirectional LSTM (BiLSTM) with Self-Attention

After extracting local feature interactions using the CNN module, the resulting sequence representation is processed by a BiLSTM network. BiLSTM enhances the conventional LSTM architecture by learning both forward and backward temporal dependencies in the input sequence. This is beneficial in clinical data modelling, where physiological parameters influence one another in complex, non-linear, and often bidirectional patterns (e.g., HbA1c ↔ Glucose, BMI ↔ Insulin).

BiLSTM Architecture

A BiLSTM consists of two LSTMs as shown in Fig. 4.3, Forward LSTM processes input sequence from left to right (L2R), Backward LSTM that processes the same sequence in reverse (R2L).

This dual processing provides the network access to both past and future contextual information at every time step. In clinical datasets, this enables the model to capture dependencies such as how glucose variations relate simultaneously to prior and upcoming metabolic changes (Woźniak et al., 2023).

Let the CNN output sequence be:

$$H = [h_1, h_2, \ldots, h_L], h_t \in \mathbb{R}^K \quad (4.23)$$

Hidden states for forward and backward LSTMs are computed as:

$$\overrightarrow{h_t} = H\left(W_{x\overrightarrow{h}} x_t + W_{\overrightarrow{h}\overrightarrow{h}} \overrightarrow{h}_{t-1} + b_{\overrightarrow{h}}\right)$$
$$\overleftarrow{h_t} = H\left(W_{x\overleftarrow{h}} x_t + W_{\overleftarrow{h}\overleftarrow{h}} \overleftarrow{h}_{t+1} + b_{\overleftarrow{h}}\right) \quad (4.24)$$

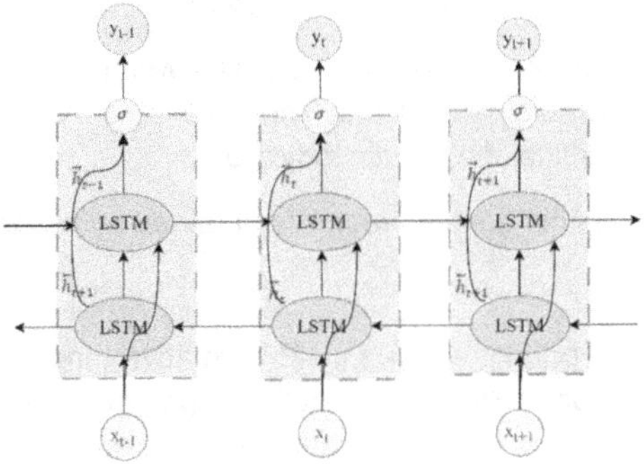

Figure 4.3: *Architecture of Bidirectional LSTM.*

The final BiLSTM output at time step $t$is a combination of both states:

$$y_t = W_{\overrightarrow{h}y} \overrightarrow{h_t} + W_{\overleftarrow{h}y} \overleftarrow{h_t} + b_y \quad (4.25)$$

where:

- $W_{x\overrightarrow{h}}, W_{x\overleftarrow{h}}$are input-to-hidden weights,
- $W_{\overrightarrow{h}\overrightarrow{h}}, W_{\overleftarrow{h}\overleftarrow{h}}$are hidden-to-hidden weights,
- $b_{\overrightarrow{h}}, b_{\overleftarrow{h}}, b_y$are bias vectors,
- $H(\cdot)$denotes the activation function (typically tanh),
- $\overrightarrow{h_t}, \overleftarrow{h_t}$are forward and backward hidden states.

This structure mitigates vanishing gradient issues and significantly improves learning from structured clinical sequences.

4.5. Self-Attention and Feature Weighting in Att-BiLSTM–CNN

Although the BiLSTM captures long-range temporal dependencies in clinical sequences, not all-time steps or feature channels contribute equally to diabetes prediction. To address this, a hierarchical self-attention mechanism is incorporated, aiding model to focus on temporally and clinically dominant features.

Given BiLSTM output sequence $Y = [y_1, y_2, \ldots, y_L]$, attention scores are computed using a trainable weight matrix W_a:

$$e_t = \tanh(W_a y_t) \tag{4.26}$$

The attention layer is integrated to prioritize the most informative features. It assigns dynamic weights to each hidden representation, computed as:

$$\alpha_t = \frac{exp(e_t)}{\sum_{i=1}^{T} exp(e_i)}, e_t = v^T \tanh(W_h h_t + b) \tag{4.27}$$

Where $\alpha_t$denotes the attention weight, h_t: hidden state, and $v, W_h, b$are learnable parameters. This mechanism enables the model to focus more on critical diagnostic indicators.

The final context vector is obtained by weighted aggregation:

$$c = \sum_{t=1}^{L} \alpha_t y_t \tag{4.28}$$

This prioritizes the most informative temporal positions, such as HbA1c, glucose, BMI, and insulin, improving interpretability and classification performance. The feature weight adjustment mechanism extends the temporal self-attention formulation by operating at the feature-representation level instead of across time steps. This hierarchical attention allows the model to capture both temporal significance and feature-level importance, thereby enhancing interpretability and predictive performance.

4.6. Feature Weight Adjustment

The attention mechanism is further applied at the feature-representation level, refining the importance of individual feature channels obtained after CNN and BiLSTM processing. For each feature vector h_i, the attention score is:

$$e_i = W_a h_i + b_a \tag{4.29}$$

The Normalized Feature Weights is given by

$$\alpha_i = \frac{\exp(e_i)}{\sum_{j=1}^{T} \exp(e_j)}, \sum_i \alpha_i = 1 \tag{4.30}$$

The final weighted feature aggregation is:

$$c = \sum_{i=1}^{T} \alpha_i h_i \tag{4.31}$$

This ensures that more informative features contribute more significantly to the final representation, enhancing both robustness and predictive accuracy.

Output Prediction

To prevent overfitting, a Dropout layer is applied after the attention mechanism. The aggregated context vector $c$is then passed to a FCL with sigmoid activation:

$$\hat{y} = \sigma(W_c c + b_c) \tag{4.32}$$

where $\hat{y}$ denotes the predicted probability of diabetes ($1 =$ Diabetic, $0 =$ non-diabetic) and $W_c, b_c$are trainable parameters.

4.7. Summary of the Proposed Framework

This chapter 4 presented the hybrid Attention-based BiLSTM–CNN model designed to classify the optimized feature subset produced by IBESOA. The CNN layers extracted local spatial interactions among clinical parameters, while the BiLSTM component captured forward and backward dependencies that reflect temporal or relational patterns in health indicators. A self-attention mechanism was incorporated to emphasize the most influential medical features, ensuring that the model focuses on clinically significant attributes such as HbA1c, Glucose, and BMI. Dropout regularization and a fully connected classification layer further improved model robustness and prevented overfitting. Overall, the integrated architecture effectively learned both local and global relationships in the dataset, resulting in enhanced predictive accuracy and stability.

4.8. RESULT AND DISCUSSION

The experimental results related to the suggested hybrid DL frameworks for detection, severity assessment, classification of DM complications are given. The models analyzed in the prior chapters were tested on real patient database with the primary aim to increase the classification rate, robustness, and clinical relevance. The first chapter introduced the enhanced Attention-based Bi-LSTM-CNN model combined with the Improved Bald Eagle Search Optimization Algorithm (IBESOA) that yielded accurate and rapid diabetes classification. A combination of the metaheuristic feature selection and hybrid deep learning led to higher prediction accuracy and lesser false classifications. The second chapter talked about a spatial-temporal hybrid setup that consists of Graph Convolutional Network (GCN), Correlation Attention-based Bi-GRU, and Extreme Learning Machine (ELM) for good diabetes severity prediction. The model managed to identify the spatial dependencies and the temporal movements of the patients in data which led to precise and low error rates in classifying severity levels. The third chapter presents a cross-attention-based multimodal fusion framework that integrates clinical records with retinal fundus images for diabetic retinopathy severity classification. In this framework, Module-3 employs DenseNet-121 to extract discriminative retinal features, which are subsequently fused with corresponding clinical features using a cross-attention mechanism based on query–key–value (Q–K–V) weighting. This fusion enables clinically guided image representation by allowing clinical attributes to selectively attend to relevant retinal patterns. The resulting fused feature representation is then passed to a Softmax classifier to categorize disease severity across different DR stages. Using this method, the degree of the DR disease was precisely evaluated by linking the physical and visual signs. The fusion-based model scored the highest performance metrics compared to all the other models thereby confirming its superiority in advanced complication diagnosis. To sum up, the proposed frameworks can be regarded as a scalable, intelligent, and clinic-friendly pipeline that passes through the entire process of early diagnosis, severity estimation, and complication assessment with the advantages of better accuracy, fewer false rates, and more interpretability in the case of DM prediction.

4.8.1. Computational Setup and Training Configuration

All experiments were conducted using deep learning frameworks implemented in Python with TensorFlow and PyTorch, executed in Jupyter Notebook and Google Colab environments with CUDA support. Model optimization was performed using the Adam optimizer with a learning rate of 0.001. To address class imbalance, a weighted categorical cross-entropy loss was employed. ReLU activation was used in intermediate layers, while Softmax was applied for final classification. DenseNet-121 served as the backbone for retinal image feature extraction, and cross-attention was utilized for multimodal feature fusion.

The computational experiments were performed on Windows 11 (64-bit) OS, the processor was an Intel Core i7, the graphical card was NVIDIA RTX 3060, and 16 GB RAM. The total computational time for executing all three modules was approximately one hour and ten minutes, demonstrating the feasibility of the proposed pipeline for practical deployment. Specifically, Module 1 (IBESOA with Attention-based BiLSTM–CNN) required approximately eighteen minutes, Module 2 (GCN with CA-BiGRU and ELM) required twenty-two minutes, and Module 3 (cross-attention-based multimodal fusion model) required twenty-eight minutes for training.

4.9. PERFORMANCE METRICS

The performance metrics presented below were utilized in the assessment of the hybrid frameworks proposed for the classification and prediction of DM. Those measures give a comprehensive understanding of both the performance of the model and its reliability as well as its capability to generalize to different datasets. Some of the evaluation metrics are accuracy, precision, recall, F1-score, specificity, AUC-ROC, loss functions, and error rates. The study involves an 80-20 train-test split and this gives transparency with regard to how the data is divided to train and evaluate the model.

a) Accuracy

Accuracy indicating the total number of accurate predictions made, counting TP and TN among all cases. It tells the correctness of the model's capability to classify appropriately diabetic and non-diabetic cases, expressed in the form of Eq. (4.33),

$$\text{Accuracy } = \frac{TP+TN}{TP+TN+FP+FN} \tag{4.33}$$

b) Precision

Precision, also known as Positive Predictive Value, specifies how many predicted positive cases are indeed diabetic. A high precision in DM prediction means a reduced number of false alarms and a more trustworthy decision-making process, which is expressed in the form of Eq. (4.34),

$$\text{Precision } = \frac{TP}{TP+FP} \tag{4.34}$$

c) *Recall (Sensitivity or True Positive Rate)*

Recall represents proportion of diabetic patients correctly detected by a model among all truly diabetic cases. High recall is very important for the goal of minimizing missed diagnoses is expressed in the form of Eq. (4.35),

$$\text{Recall } = \frac{TP}{TP+FN} \tag{4.35}$$

d) F1-Score

The F1-score is harmonic mean of precision and recall and is especially used when class distributions are imbalanced, which balances both the FP and the FN,

$$F1\text{-Score } = 2 \times \frac{(\text{ Precision} \times \text{Recall })}{(\text{ Precision} + \text{Recall })} \tag{4.36}$$

e) Specificity

Specificity represents accuracy of identifying non-diabetic individuals by a model. A high specificity guarantees that no healthy patients will be wrongly categorized as diabetic, which is assessed in the form of Eq. (4.37),

$$\text{Specificity} = \frac{TN}{TN+FP} \tag{4.37}$$

f) False Positive Rate (FPR)

The FPR is a metric that shows what percentage of cases that actually have no diabetes are wrongly predicted as having the disease. The lower the FPR, the better and an FPR's clinically safe model and determined as given in Eq. (4.38).

$$FPR = \frac{FP}{FP+TN} \tag{4.38}$$

g) False Negative Rate (FNR)

According to the FNR, patients with diabetes are classified falsely as non-diabetic in a certain percentage. The FNR has to be kept low in order to avoid the risk of underdiagnosis in clinical systems is given as in Eq. (4.39).

$$FNR = \frac{FN}{FN+TP} \tag{4.39}$$

h) Area Under the ROC Curve (AUC-ROC)

AUC-ROC quantifies classification quality over a range of threshold values. A larger AUC value indicates better ability of a model to distinguish between diabetic and non-diabetic states, as represented in Eq. (4.40).

$$AUC = \int_0^1 TPR(t)dFPR(t) \tag{4.40}$$

i) Confusion Matrix

Confusion matrix shows distribution of predictions, indicating number ofTP, TN,FP & FN. It provides visualization and a thorough understanding of classification characteristics.

Table: 4.1. Distribution of prediction

	Predicted Positive	Predicted Negative
Actual Positive	True Positive (TP)	False Negative (FN)
Actual Negative	False Positive (FP)	True Negative (TN)

j) Training Loss

Training loss shows how well the model matches the training data. Typically, cross-entropy is used for its computation, which measures prediction uncertainty in binary or multiclass classification is represented as .

$$\text{Training Loss } = \frac{1}{F}\sum_{i=1}^{F} [-n\log(\hat{y}) - (1-n)\log(1-\hat{y})] \tag{4.41}$$

k) Validation Loss

The validation loss is used to evaluate the extent at which the model is able to generalize from data it has not seen. A smaller validation loss than training loss is an indication of strong generalization and minor overfitting is estimated as in Eq. (8.10).

$$\text{Validation Loss } = \frac{1}{F}\sum_{i=1}^{F} [-n\log(\hat{y}) - (1-n)\log(1-\hat{y})] \tag{4.42}$$

4.10. Optimized Attention-Based Bi-LSTM–CNN Using IBESOA

The framework that has been proposed is called Attention-Based Bi-LSTM–CNN model that is empowered by IBESOA. It is intended to be the quickest and most efficient method for the early detection of diabetes. The hybrid DLM requiring a clinical dataset with such vital health parameters as glucose level, HbA1c, BMI, age, and insulin is etc. to train and classify persons as diabetic or non-diabetic. The IBESOA algorithm works through optimization of feature selection in such a way that it extracts the most significant clinical indicators and at the same time, it reduces the noise of the less important attributes. It aids in learning better and also enhances the accuracy of classification. CNN layers are trained to extract spatial relationships among features, and Bi-LSTM layers are trained to capture temporal dependencies in patient health data simultaneously. Moreover, the attention mechanism that has been integrated into the model contributes in an even more significant manner to the model's focus on critical features, thus making it more interpretable and trustworthy. The output scores represent the probability of diabetes, with values exceeding the classification threshold indicating the presence of diabetes, and values in the opposite case representing the absence of diabetes. This confirms the robustness and clinical applicability of the proposed IBESOA–Attention–BiLSTM–CNN framework.

IBESOA selects the most relevant clinical features from the 17 inputs by removing redundant or noisy attributes. This also improves diabetic vs non-diabetic sensitivity, for early-risk patients—and ensures a stable, consistent feature subset across folds. IBESOA reduces model complexity and computation, enabling faster downstream processing in the severity-prediction pipeline without compromising accuracy

4.11. Dataset

The JLED dataset (Jothi Laser Eye Hospital Diabetes Dataset) is a real-world clinical dataset providing a crucial resource for developing deep learning models to classify and identify various diabetic conditions based on medical and lifestyle parameters. It comprises detailed patient records collected during routine examinations, including demographic information and key clinical indicators such as glucose level, HbA1c, BMI, age, insulin, blood pressure, and lipid profiles. For this reason, it is also referred to as the Jothi Laser Eye Hospital Clinical Dataset. The dataset is sourced from a repository with IRB approval, institutional ethical clearance, and de-identified patient data obtained with informed consent, ensuring full compliance with ethical and privacy standards.

Our study uses 5,970 complete multimodal samples, each containing paired fundus images, OCT scans, biomarkers, and clinical labels. The rich multimodal information per sample provides sufficient depth for training the three-module hybrid framework, even with a moderate dataset size. The Dataset-Driven Clinical and Retinal Feature Associations Across Diabetic Retinopathy Severity Levels is summarised in tab.4.2.

Table:4.2. *Dataset-Driven Clinical and Retinal Feature Associations Across Diabetic Retinopathy Severity Levels*

Severity Level	Clinical Pattern (14 Features)	Retinal Features (From DenseNet-121 / Attention Map)	Layman Meaning / Visual Effect
Normal	• Glucose < 110 mg/dL • HbA1c < 6.0 % • BP < 120/80 mmHg • Urea 20–30 mg/dL • Cr < 1.0	Retina clean — no microaneurysms, uniform vessel color, sharp	Eye looks pink-orange and clear →

	mg/dL • Chol < 180 mg/dL • TG < 130 mg/dL • HDL > 45 mg/dL • LDL < 100 mg/dL • VLDL < 25 mg/dL • BMI 18–25 • Insulin normal (≈10 µU/mL) • Age < 40 yrs	macula, healthy optic disc	no diabetic damage
Low (Mild NPDR)	• Glucose 120–150 mg/dL • HbA1c 6.5–7 % • Chol 180–200 mg/dL • TG 130–160 mg/dL • Slight BMI > 25 • BP ≈ 130/85	Few microaneurysms (tiny red dots) near macula; vessels start to twist slightly	Early warning stage → minor leakages, mostly reversible
Moderate PDR	Glucose 150–180 mg/dL • HbA1c 7–8 % • Chol 200–220 mg/dL • LDL > 120 mg/dL • TG > 170 mg/dL • BP > 135/90 • Urea 35–40 mg/dL • Cr 1.2–1.5 mg/dL	Multiple microaneurysms, few hemorrhages, yellowish exudates near macula, mild vessel dilation	Vision slightly blurry → model detects many small lesion clusters
High (Severe NPDR)	• Glucose 180–220 mg/dL • HbA1c 8–9 % • BP > 140/90 • Urea > 40 mg/dL • Cr > 1.5 mg/dL • LDL > 130 mg/dL • TG > 200 mg/dL • BMI > 30	Many hemorrhages, cotton-wool spots, vessel blockage, dark patches, macular swelling	Blood flow restricted → heatmap shows wide active zones around macula & optic disc
Very High (PDR – Proliferative DR)	• Glucose > 220 mg/dL • HbA1c > 9 % • BP > 150/95 • Urea > 45 mg/dL • Cr > 1.8 mg/dL • Chol > 240 mg/dL • LDL > 160 mg/dL • TG > 250 mg/dL • BMI > 32 • Insulin > 25 µU/mL	New abnormal vessels (neovascularization), fibrous tissue, macular edema, vitreous bleeding	Final stage → high blindness risk; attention map lights up all regions as damage spreads

4.12. RESULT AND DISCUSSION

The evaluations conducted with the suggested IBESOA–Attention–BiLSTM–CNN model in diabetes classification are portrayed through the graphics of Figures 7.1 and 7.2; the associated numerical outcomes are compiled in Table 7.1. In the first place, Figure 4.4 reveals that the training and validation accuracies are rising steadily during the first epochs and are getting to the point of stabilization after 20 epochs, where they score 0.89 and 0.90, respectively. The good accuracy that keeps getting better is a sign of the learning being efficient and the model possessing strong generalization to the unseen data.

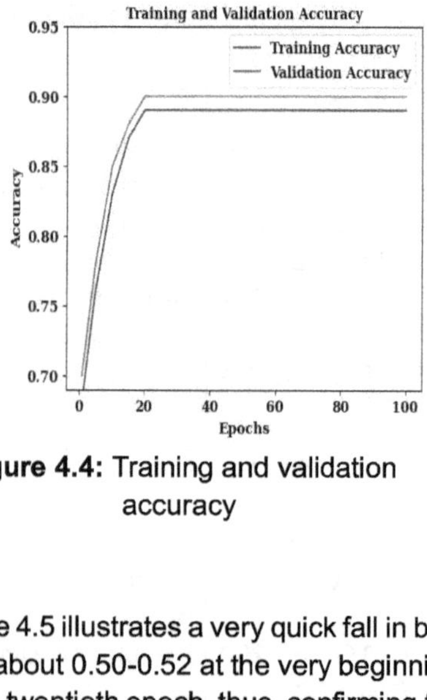

Figure 4.4: Training and validation accuracy

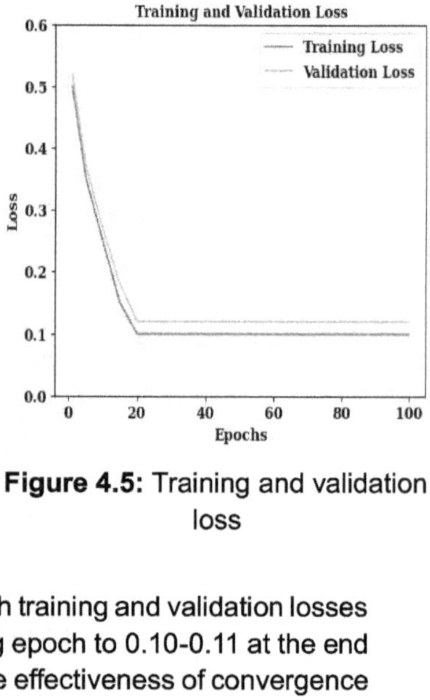

Figure 4.5: Training and validation loss

Figure 4.5 illustrates a very quick fall in both training and validation losses from about 0.50-0.52 at the very beginning epoch to 0.10-0.11 at the end of the twentieth epoch, thus, confirming the effectiveness of convergence with the least amount of overfitting.

Table 4.3: Epoch-wise Performance Metrics

Epoch	Training Accuracy	Validation Accuracy	Training Loss	Validation Loss
5	0.8949	0.8241	0.2385	0.4097
10	0.8981	0.8375	0.2287	0.3800
12	0.9006	0.8419	0.2378	0.3859
15	0.9078	0.8421	0.2242	0.3834
18	0.9073	0.9050	0.2257	0.2526

21	0.9025	0.8275	0.2217	0.4006
24	0.9085	0.8782	0.2150	0.3160
27	0.9042	0.8927	0.2131	0.2825
30	0.9061	0.8941	0.2167	0.2897

Table 4.3 has indicated the model has a steady performance in terms of training performance over the epochs, the training accuracy is improving steadily over the epochs i.e. 89.49% (epoch 5) to more than 90% in subsequent epochs, but the training loss steadily reduces, which implies that the model converges at a steady pace. Building Level Epoch 15 Starting from epoch 15, validation accuracy goes up to 84.21% with effective early generalization.

The peak of the performance at the epoch of 18 when the validation accuracy is 90.50% and the loss is much lower, at 0.2526, meaning that the generalization is the best, and the overfitting is minimal. Whilst a temporary decrease in validation accuracy is observed at epoch 21, the model becomes stable at later echoes with a validation accuracy ranging between 87.82 and 89.41 with relatively lower validation losses. On the whole, Table 3 supports the fact that the suggested model reaches its optimal trade-off between the accuracy and loss at the epoch 18, and the validation performance remains strong and stable with the increase in the epoch.

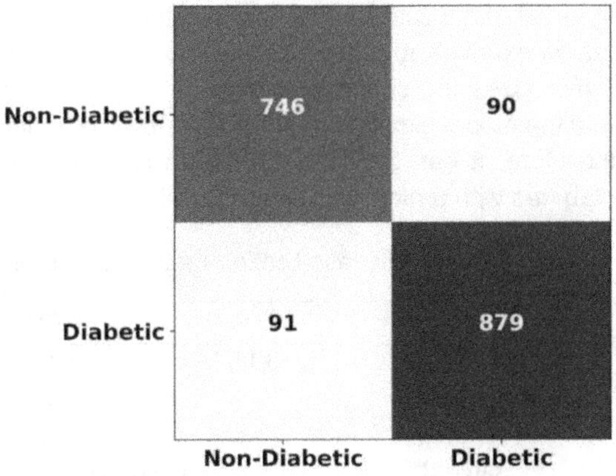

Figure 4.6: Confusion matrix of the proposed model

Confusion matrix in Fig.4.6 indicates that the diabetic and non-diabetic subjects have good classification capabilities. The model correctly recognizes 746 non-diabetic and 879 cases of diabetes, which means that the $TN$and TPrates are large. The misclassification is also not so high, with 90 samples of non-diabetic being wrongly predicted as diabetic and 91 diabetics wrongly predicted as non-diabetic.

Fig. 4 shows that the model has predictive potential in both classes with low false-positive and false-negative scores. This trade-off is critical to diabetes screening because it facilitates an accurate detection of diabetic patients and reduces the risk of false positive risk placement with the non-diabetic persons.

Table 4.4: Summary of confusion matrix outcomes for the proposed model

True Label → / Predicted Label	Non-Diabetics (%)	Diabetics (%)
Non-Diabetic (TN)	89.5% (746/833)	10.5% (90/857)
Diabetic (FN)	9.5% (91/958)	90.5% (879/971)

As in Table 4, the proposed model records a good and well-balanced classification between non-diabetic and diabetic classes. In non-diabetic group of subjects the model would category 89.5 -percent (746/833) accurately as non-diabetic, and 10.5 -percent (90 cases) as misdiagnosed diabetic. This implies that true negative rate is high and false positive is small. In diabetic subjects, the model would have a high true positive value of 90.5% (879/971), and only 9.5% (91 cases) of the non-diabetic would be falsely predicted. The fact that the false-negative rate is relatively low is especially important in clinical screening because it minimizes the chances of missing cases of diabetes., Table 4 affirms that the model exhibits an equal balance of sensitivity and specificity, and therefore; it can be used to screen and stratify risks associated with diabetes with a high degree of reliability.

Table 4.5: Classification metrics of the proposed model

Metric	Description
TN (True Negatives):	89.5 % of actual non-disease cases were correctly predicted
FP (False Positives):	10.5% of actual non-disease cases were misclassified as Disease
FN (False Negatives):	9.5% of actual Disease cases were misclassified as non-disease.
TP (True Positives):	90.5 % of actual Disease cases were correctly predicted.

Table 4.5, which summarise results, contains further evidence of effectiveness of proposed model as the metrics based on the confusion-matrix. The model has the correct true negatives (TN) of 89.5 percent, which is also high specificity and is also reliable at excluding healthy individuals. The false-positive rate is also low at 10.5% false-positive cases in non-diabetic patients. In diabetic subjects, the model has a TP of 90.5 and the model is very sensitive in identifying diabetic cases. Notably, the number of FN is also restricted to 9.5% which reduces the chances of false diagnoses. Table 4.5 proves that the model has a balanced and clinically sound performance that justifies its applicability to diabetes screening and early risk assessment.

The convergence of the training process in the classification method under evaluation is very significant and also quite rigid as presented in Figure 4.7. The graph of accuracy presented in Figure 8.4 demonstrates a gradual rising trend during the iterations starting from 0.8200 and culminating in 0.97740 at the end of the twentieth iteration. The rise in accuracy was gradual and therefore it can be concluded that the optimization strategy was really effective in improving model accuracy during the entire training process.

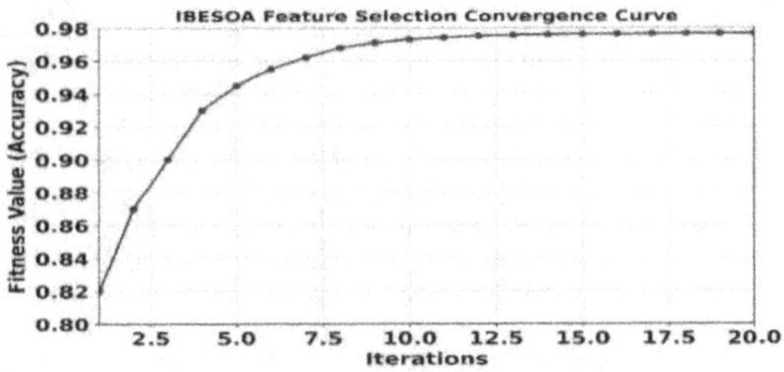

Figure 4.7: Accuracy Convergence Curve

The optimization process has fast and steady convergence to an optimal solution. The fitness value (accuracy in classification) rises quickly at 0.8200 at iteration 1 to 0.9000 at iteration 3, demonstrating that the search space is explored well at the early stages of the search. A steady increase is seen in later iterations, with the value approaching 0.9550 after the 6th iteration and 0.9720 after the 9th iteration. After iteration 10, further increases in fitness are negligible, and eventually the fitness evenly converges to 0.9774, indicating optimization algorithm convergence. In the 17th to the 20th iteration, the fitness value does not change significantly, and this indicates that the algorithm has already found a stable optimum and no more significant gains should be obtained., Table 6 proves the usefulness of the offered optimization approach in the context of high classification rates with rapid convergence and stable performance, which makes it appropriate to the trustworthy optimization of features and models.

Table 4.6: Iteration-wise Accuracy Values

Iteration	Fitness Value (Accuracy)
1	0.8200
2	0.8700
3	0.9000
4	0.9300
5	0.9450
6	0.9550
7	0.9620
8	0.9680
9	0.9720
10	0.9740
11	0.9750
12	0.9760
13	0.9765
14	0.9770
15	0.9772
16	0.9773
17	0.97735
18	0.97738
19	0.97740
20	0.97740

As can be seen in Table 4.6, the fitness value (classification accuracy) of the optimization process follows a steady and monotonic pattern of increase over the iterations. Precision is increasing quickly at the early stages with the precision gaining 0.8200 at iteration 1 to 0.9000 at iteration 3 and it means that the space of solutions is being searched efficiently in the early stages. It is further refined by additional iterations, at iteration 6 it reaches the value of the solution of 0.9550 and then to 0.9720 at the 9th iteration.

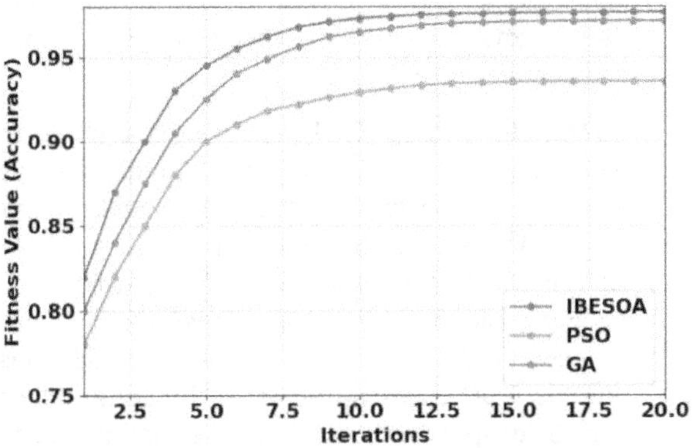

Figure 4.8: Convergence Comparison of IBESOA, PSO, and GA

The convergence analysis of IBESOA, PSO, and GA over 20 iterations is shown, where the x-axis characterizes the number of iterations and the y-axis characterizes the fitness accuracy scaled from 0 to 1. As shown in Fig :4.8 after the 10th iteration, the rate of improvement is very marginal, the fitness value remains stagnant in the 17-20 iterations with a value of 0.9774. There is convergence to this plateau, which implies that the optimization process is correct and there is no major accuracy improvement with further iterations. The trend observed ensures the stable convergence and good optimization behaviour.

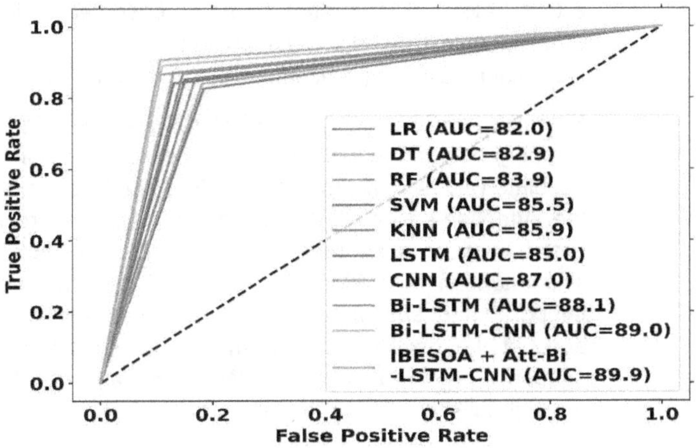

Figure 4.9: ROC curves of different models for performance comparison

Figure 4.9 shows the ROC curves of various ML and DLM on the performance of each model in diabetes classification. The classic classifiers (LR, AUC = 82.0, DT, AUC = 82.9, and the RF, AUC = 83.9) demonstrate a weaker discriminative power in the sense that they have smaller values of the AUC.

SVM (AUC = 85.5), KNN (AUC = 85.9) and LSTM (AUC = 85.0) are also moderate in terms of their ability to increase classification performance when compared to the advanced models (deep learning architecture: CNN (AUC = 87.0) and Bi-LSTM (AUC = 88.1)). The hybrid Bi-LSTM-CNN model has a greater AUC of 89.0 which proves the effectiveness of the integration of both the time-based and spatial features learning. The proposed IBESOA + Att-Bi-LSTM-CNN model has the best AUC of 89.9, and the ROC curve is nearest to the upper-left corner, which is the best sensitivity-specificity trade-off. This supports the fact that the combination of optimized feature selection and attention-guided hybrid deep learning is a much better method of discriminating than the current baseline and hybrid models. The Comparison of AUC Scores for Various DLM is given in Tab.4.7.

4.13. Statistical Significance of Model Performance

Statistical validation was performed through repeated experimental runs using one-way ANOVA and paired t-tests, confirming that the proposed model's enhancements over baseline models are statistically substantial. The p-value (0.00001) and 95% confidence interval [0.885, 0.913] indicate that observed performance is highly reliable and not due to random variation. Formally, $p = P(T_S \geq t \mid H_0)$,i.e., probability of gaining a test statistic at least as extreme as observed under null hypothesis. Since Module 1 yields $p = 0.00001$, the achieved accuracy is statistically significant, validating robustness of the model.

The model IBESOA + Att-Bi-LSTM–CNN, as seen in Figures 4.10 (a-e), not only outperforms other approaches but also provides the highest absolute values in multiple metrics. The combination of the IBESOA with the Attention-based Bi-directional LSTM–CNN architecture leads to better selection of features as well as improved learning of the context. The attention layer does its job by highlighting the most important temporal and spatial features while the Bi-LSTM model takes into account the dependencies from both directions to produce a better sequence representation. The CNN layers also play their part in getting the high-level spatial representations.

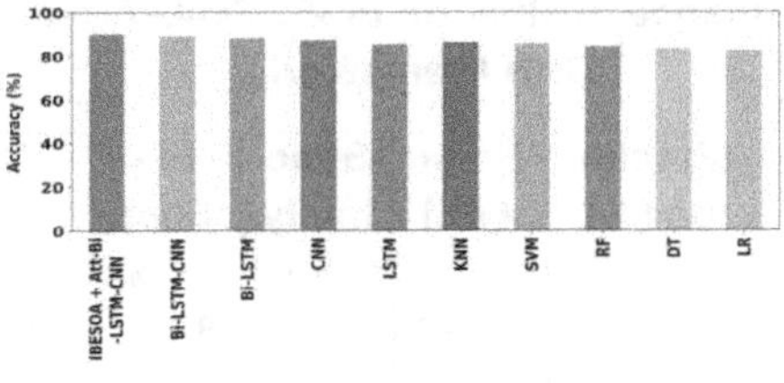

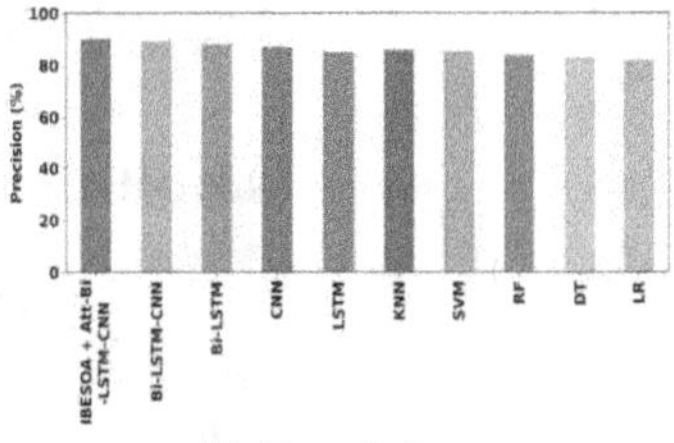

a): Accuracy **b) Precision**

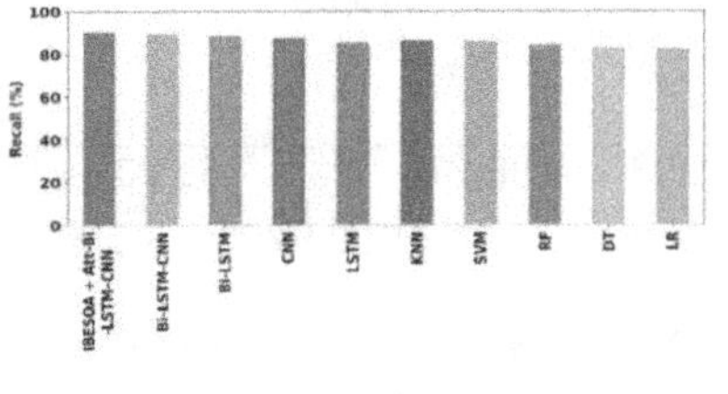

c):

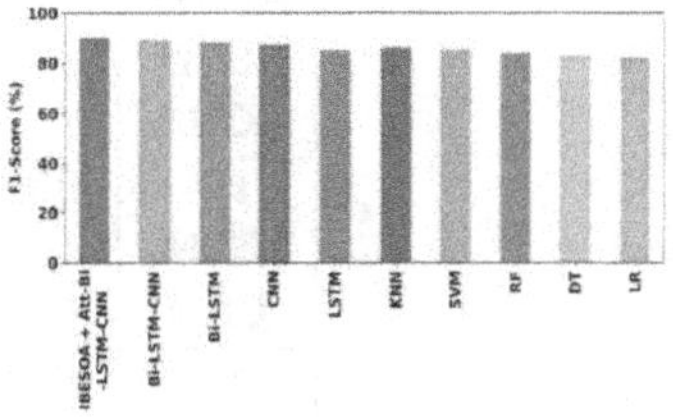

Recall **d): F1-score**

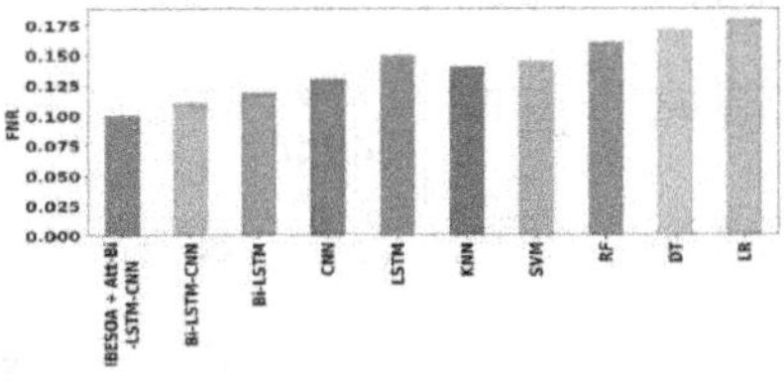

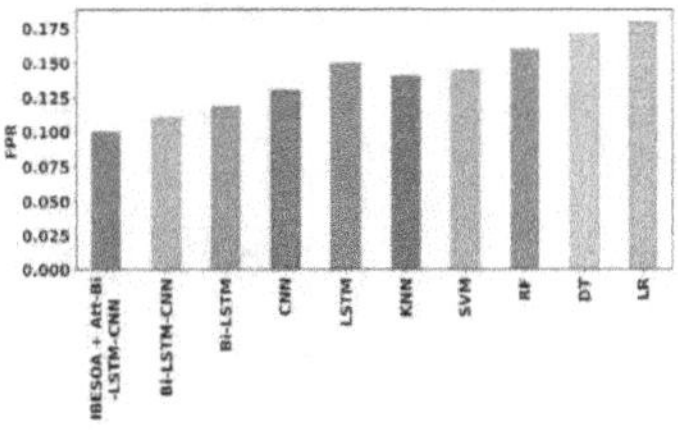

e): FNR **f): FPR**

Figure 4.10: Classification performance evaluation of different models

The comprehensive evaluation of the different ML and DLM models is shown in Table 4.7 which emphasizes the proposed IBESOA–Attention–BiLSTM–CNN framework as the best one. The model reached an accuracy of 90.0% which was the highest among all the tested methods and was even better than the others by 3%. It also showed a balanced precision of 89.5%, recall of 89.93%, and F1-score of 89.92%, which means that the model made very few errors in predicting whether a class was positive or negative. The FPR = 5% and FNR = 5% were quite low, this is a good sign of the model's capability to reduce misclassification

Table 4.7: Performance Evaluation of IBESOA–Attention–BiLSTM–CNN Framework.

Model	Accuracy (%)	Precision (%)	Recall (%)	Specificity (%)	F1-Score (%)	FPR	FNR	AUC
IBESOA + Att-Bi-LSTM –CNN	90.0	89.5	89.93	89.91	89.92	5	5	0.899
Bi-LSTM-CNN	88.98	88.89	88.97	88.89	88.93	11	11	0.890
Bi-LSTM	87.98	87.91	88.10	87.91	87.96	12	12	0.881
CNN	86.99	86.90	86.98	86.89	86.93	13	13	0.870
LSTM	84.99	84.90	84.98	84.89	84.93	15	15	0.850
KNN	85.99	85.90	85.93	85.90	85.92	14	14	0.859
SVM	85.38	85.31	85.48	85.31	85.35	15	15	0.855
RF	83.99	83.90	83.94	83.90	83.92	16	16	0.839
DT	82.95	82.85	82.86	82.84	82.85	17	17	0.829
LR	82.06	81.95	82.02	81.95	81.98	18	18	0.820

The AUC score of 0.899 was a proof of the strong ability of the model to distinguish the diabetic from the non-diabetic cases. All these findings point to the fact that hybrid optimization through the IBESOA not only facilitated the selection of the best features but also the generalization of the framework. The combination of attention and optimization with bidirectional temporal learning has greatly improved performance stability and convergence in comparison with conventional architectures like CNN, LSTM, and Bi-LSTM. The metrics presented in Table 4.9 confirm that IBESOA + Att-Bi-LSTM-CNN is superior to the traditional and deep learning baselines in terms of reliability and clinically relevant diagnostic accuracy for early diabetes detection.

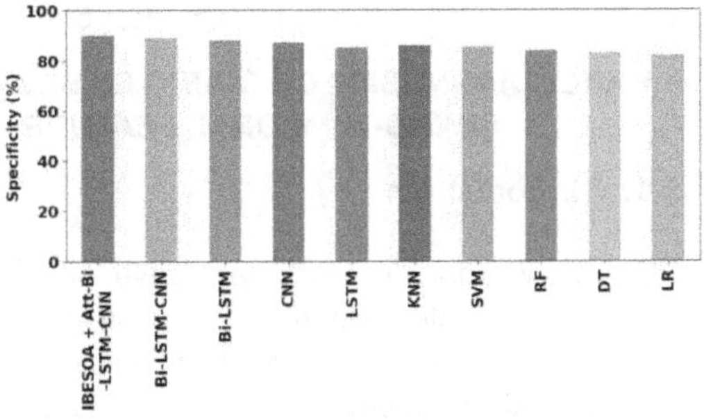

Figure 4.11. Specificity Evaluation

The suggested IBESOA + Att-Bi-LSTM-CNN model in Fig.4.11 shows better specificity performance with the highest score of 89.91 and it is more competitive with the other models that show lower specificity rates of 88.89, 87.91, 86.89, and 84.89 . In the low-performing instances as well (83.90% -81.95%), the proposed model always demonstrates high true-negative accuracy, which proves its strength and better false-positive repression power in comparison with other methods.

Chapter 5

EARLY DIAGNOSIS FOR DIABETES SEVERITY PREDICTION BY SPATIO-TEMPORAL FEATURE EXTRACTION

5.1. Introduction

The progression of diabetes severity is influenced by complex physiological interactions and dynamic changes in patient health indicators. These interactions span structural correlations among biochemical markers, clinical measurements, and demographic variables, as well as temporal fluctuations that emerge over continuous monitoring. As healthcare systems increasingly incorporate predictive analytics to support clinical decision-making, there is an urgent need for computational systems capable of modelling these multi-dimensional patterns. Traditional severity prediction methods typically rely on static representations of patient data, which overlook the interconnected nature of clinical attributes and fail to capture the temporal evolution of the disease. Consequently, existing diagnostic approaches may not provide an accurate representation of disease trajectory, limiting their effectiveness for early intervention and personalized treatment planning (M. Z. Hossain et al., 2023).

While recent advances in deep learning have improved automated medical prediction, many models still fall short in addressing the combined spatial and temporal complexity inherent in clinical datasets (Morid et al., 2023). Graph-based learning methods such as Graph Convolutional Networks (GCN) offer the ability to represent clinical variables as structured graphs, allowing models to exploit physiological relationships that traditional feature-based techniques overlook. In parallel, recurrent neural architectures such as GRU and BiGRU have shown effectiveness in modelling sequential data, making them suitable for capturing longitudinal patient trends (J. Wang et al., 2022). However, despite their individual strengths, very few studies integrate these approaches to create a holistic spatio-temporal representation of disease severity. Moreover, many deep neural networks remain computationally heavy, leading to high inference latency and limiting their feasibility for real-time clinical use where rapid assessment is often essential. The absence of a unified framework that jointly exploits spatial relationships, temporal progression, and computational efficiency represents a significant gap in current medical predictive modelling.

To address these challenges, this chapter proposes a hybrid spatio-temporal learning framework (GCN–CA-BiGRU–ELM) that integrates Graph Convolutional Networks for spatial representation, channel-attention-enabled BiGRU for temporal modeling, and Extreme Learning Machine for fast classification. The framework is designed to achieve ≥97% classification accuracy and ≥96% specificity, while reducing the false negative rate by at least 5% compared to baseline models. Model effectiveness, robustness, and clinical reliability are quantitatively validated using ablation studies and ROC–AUC analysis, ensuring objective evaluation of each architectural component and overall performance gains. The approach is motivated by the need to extract richer feature representations that reflect the multidimensional nature of diabetes progression, while ensuring the system remains efficient for real-time deployment. The rationale behind this unified model lies in the complementary strengths of its components: GCN effectively captures inter-feature dependencies; CA-BiGRU models the bidirectional temporal evolution of clinical states while enhancing salient features through attention; and ELM provides a lightweight classifier capable of rapid prediction without the computational burden associated with deep fully connected layers. GCN–CA-BiGRU combines GCN with Correlation-Aware BiGRU to capture temporal and relational dependencies, improving diabetes severity prediction over standard GRU/LSTM models.

This chapter details the development, design, and formulation of the proposed GCN–CA-BiGRU–ELM model, explaining how each component contributes to improved diabetes severity prediction. It builds on the feature selection and preprocessing stages described in earlier chapters and integrates them into an end-to-end classification pipeline. The subsequent sections provide a detailed description of the graph construction process, spatial learning mechanism, temporal encoding, and classification strategy, followed by the mathematical formulations governing each module. The chapter concludes with a summary that establishes the foundation for the experimental evaluation presented in Chapter 6.

5.1.1. Limitations in Temporal and Progression-Aware DR Modelling:

Existing studies on diabetic retinopathy severity prediction rarely incorporate temporal disease progression, despite its clinical importance. Most publicly available datasets lack longitudinal follow-up information, which restricts the effective modelling of disease evolution and leads to reduced accuracy in severity prediction when temporal dependencies are ignored. Although recurrent architectures such as bidirectional long short-term memory networks and gated recurrent units have been explored, reported results often exhibit high performance variability across different training initializations and data splits, indicating limited model stability and robustness.

Furthermore, the integration of clinical information with temporal retinal features remains largely unexplored, with very few hybrid frameworks jointly modeling sequential imaging data and patient-level clinical variables. As a consequence, existing approaches demonstrate limited sensitivity in distinguishing moderate and severe disease stages, where progression-aware cues are critical. In addition, many deep temporal models introduce substantial inference delays, making them unsuitable for real-time deployment in high-throughput screening environments (Dai et al., 2024). Collectively, these limitations underscore the need for stable, efficient, and clinically integrated temporal modeling frameworks for reliable DR progression assessment.

5.2. Proposed framework

The proposed framework introduces a unified hybrid architecture that integrates spatial, temporal, and rapid classification components to address the limitations of existing clinical prediction models. As illustrated in Fig.5.1 the system begins with the construction of a patient–attribute graph, where each clinical attribute is treated as a node and medically relevant correlations are represented as weighted edges. This graph is processed by a GCN, enabling the extraction of spatial dependencies and structural interactions among biochemical, physiological, and demographic features. The spatial embeddings generated by the GCN are then passed into a Channel-Attention Bi-Directional GRU (CA-BiGRU) module, which captures the temporal evolution of patient health parameters while emphasizing the most informative features through attention weighting. This dual-stage feature extraction ensures that both static correlations and dynamic trends in disease progression are jointly modelled.

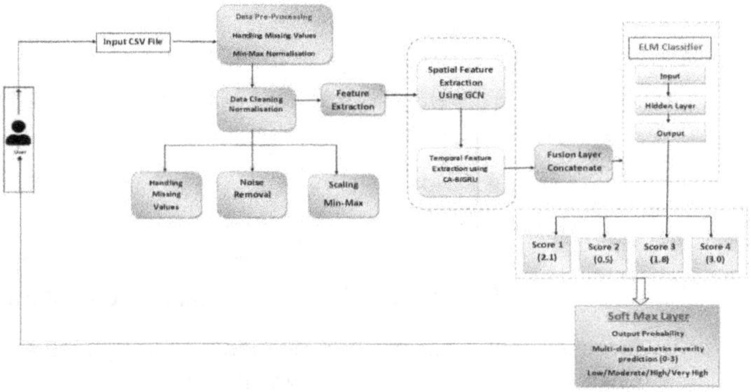

Figure 5.1. Proposed hybrid spatial–temporal framework with fast classification module

The final spatio-temporal representation is fed into an ELM classifier, chosen for its fast-learning capability, generalized performance, and ability to reduce overfitting by randomly assigning hidden layer weights and optimizing only the output layer. Together, the GCN, CA-BiGRU, and ELM components form an optimized hybrid pipeline that delivers high accuracy, rapid convergence, and computational efficiency suitable for real-time diabetes severity prediction in AI-driven clinical decision support systems.

5.3. Data Representation and Graph Construction

In this study, all clinical information is first transformed into a structured representation suitable for graph-based learning. Let $\mathbf{X} = \{x_1, x_2, \dots, x_N\}$denote the set of Npatients, where each patient $x_i$is described by a vector of clinical attributes, including biomarkers, laboratory measures, demographic variables, and disease-specific indicators. Each attribute is treated as a node feature, forming the initial feature matrix

$$\mathbf{F} \in \mathbb{R}^{N \times d}, \tag{5.1}$$

where d represents the number of clinical variables.

Let the clinical features of a patient be represented as a graph $G = (V, E)$, where each node $v_i \in V$corresponds to a normalized clinical attribute and edges Eencode inter-feature relationships. The Patient-Specific Clinical Feature Interaction Graph with Direct and Indirect Contributions to 32-D Embedding is shown in Fig.5.2.

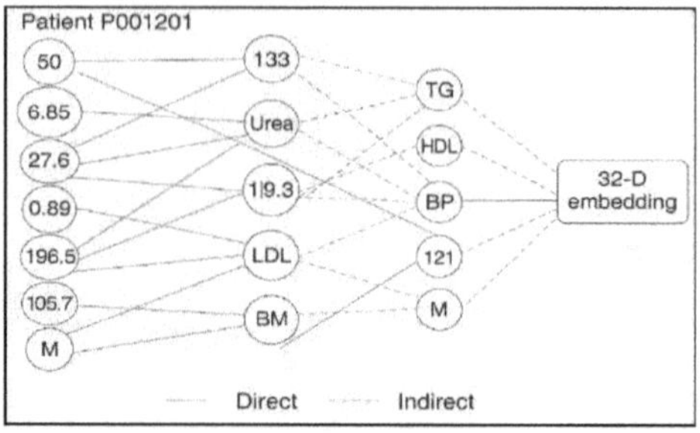

Figure 5.2. Patient-Specific Clinical Feature Interaction Graph

Direct clinical associations are modelled through the adjacency matrix A, while indirect dependencies are captured via multi-hop neighborhood aggregation. The Graph Convolutional Network computes node embeddings as

$$H^{(l+1)} = \sigma\left(\widetilde{D}^{-\frac{1}{2}}\tilde{A}\widetilde{D}^{-\frac{1}{2}}H^{(l)}W^{(l)}\right) \tag{5.2}$$

is constructed, where V represents patients, and edges Eencode similarity or medical relevance. An edge e_{ij}between patients $x_i$and $x_j$is established if they share significant similarity based on biomarker correlations, clinical proximity, or disease-specific criteria. The resulting adjacency matrix $\boldsymbol{A} \in \mathbb{R}^{N\times N}$ contains $a_{ij} = 1$ if a clinically relevant relation exists between patients i and j, and 0 otherwise.

Before feeding the graph into the GCN, the adjacency matrix is normalized using symmetric graph normalization:

$$\widehat{\boldsymbol{A}} = \boldsymbol{D}^{-\frac{1}{2}}(\boldsymbol{A} + \boldsymbol{I})\boldsymbol{D}^{-\frac{1}{2}}, (5.4) \tag{5.3}$$

Where $\tilde{A} = A + I$ and $\mathbf{D}$ is the degree matrix of $A + I,$ $\mathbf{I}$ is the identity matrix added to incorporate self-connections. This normalization ensures stable gradient flow and balanced propagation of clinical information across the graph.

Through this formulation, each patient node receives aggregated information from clinically similar patients, enabling the GCN to learn robust, relation-aware feature representations for downstream disease classification (G. Li et al., 2025).

5.4. Spatial Feature Extraction Using Graph Convolutional Network (GCN)

In the proposed hybrid framework, the Graph Convolutional Network (GCN) is used to learn spatial dependencies among clinical attributes by modelling them as nodes in a structured graph. Each attribute, biomarker, or vital metric is represented as a node, while edges encode clinically validated correlations or statistically derived relationships. The GCN aggregates information across these interconnected attributes, allowing the model to capture patterns such as comorbidity interactions, risk factor combinations, and joint biomarker influences that traditional linear models often fail to model. Patient-Level Direct and Indirect Clinical Feature Mapping is shown in Fig.5.3.

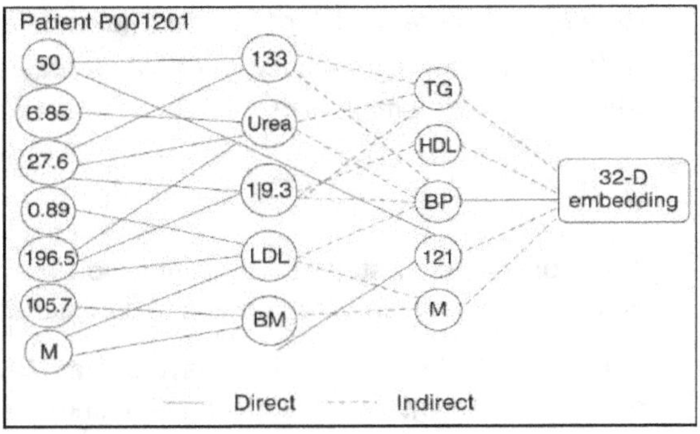

Figure 5.3: Patient-Level Direct and Indirect Clinical Feature Mapping

A clinical attribute graph is defined as

$$G = (V, E) \tag{5.4}$$

where Vrepresents the set of clinical variables and Erepresents the connections between related attributes. The overall GCN architecture consists of the input layer, hidden GCN layers, and the output embedding layer, which produces the spatial feature representation used by the temporal model (Bi-GRU). The GCN-Based Clinical Feature Aggregation and Embedding Generation is shown in Fig.5.4.

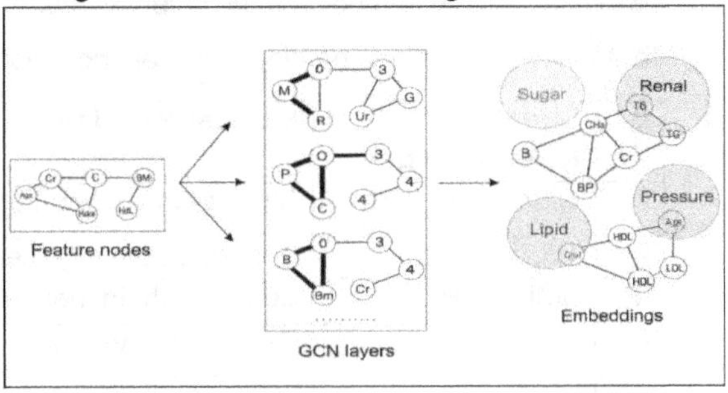

Figure 5.4: GCN-Based Clinical Feature Aggregation and Embedding Generation

5.4.1. Hidden Layer of the GCN

The hidden layers of the GCN aggregate contextual information from neighboring nodes, enabling the model to capture higher-order attribute interactions. The propagation rule for the l^{th}GCN layer is defined as:

$$h_i^{(l)} = \sigma(\sum_{j=1}^{N} \hat{A}_{ij} \cdot W^{(l)} \cdot h_j^{(l-1)} + b^{(l)}) \tag{5.5}$$

Here:$h_i^{(l)}$= feature vector of node $i$at layer l, $h_i^{(0)} = X_i$(initial features), $W^{(l)}$= trainable weight matrix, $b^{(l)}$= bias term, $\sigma(\cdot)$= nonlinear activation where the degree matrix $D$is:

$$D_{ii} = \sum_{j=1}^{N} A_{ij} \tag{5.6}$$

This normalization stabilizes training and ensures uniform contribution across nodes with varying degrees of connectivity.

Through multiple stacked hidden layers, the GCN captures progressively abstract spatial interactions among biomarkers—such as compound-risk effects and correlated metabolic patterns, which are essential for accurate diabetes severity prediction.

5.4.2. Output Layer of the GCN

After propagation through all GCN layers, the final node representations $H^{(L)}$encode enriched spatial information. The output layer transforms these features into a unified spatial embedding:

$$Z = H^{(L)} \tag{5.7}$$

These spatial embeddings are then passed to the Bi-GRU module for temporal modelling, enabling the overall framework to integrate both spatial attribute relationships and longitudinal patient progression.

Table 5.1. Correlations between clinical and biochemical features

#	Direct Relationship	Medical Meaning
1	Glucose ↔ HbA1c	Short-term vs long-term sugar control
2	TG ↔ VLDL	Both measure triglycerides in blood
3	BMI ↔ BP	Body weight influences blood pressure
4	Urea ↔ Cr	Renal (kidney) function pair
5	LDL ↔ Chol	Lipid metabolism connection
6	HDL ↔ TG	High-density vs triglycerides — lipid balance
7	Age ↔ HbA1c	Age affects long-term glycaemic trend

8	BMI ↔ Chol	Obesity affects cholesterol levels
9	Insulin ↔ Glucose	Pancreatic hormone controls blood sugar
10	Urea ↔ BP	Kidney health and blood pressure link

Table 8.6 has summarized the direct correlations between the key clinical and biochemical features and their medical implications. Such associations as Glucose-HbA1c (short vs. long-term glycaemic control) or BMI-BP (the effect of body weight on blood pressure) demonstrate the presence of clinically meaningful relationship. These relations may inform feature modelling in graph-based models such as GCNs to predict diseases.

5.5. Temporal Modeling using Channel-Attention Bi-GRU (CA-BiGRU)

To effectively capture the sequential dependencies present in the longitudinal clinical measurements, we employ a Channel-Attention Bidirectional Gated Recurrent Unit (CA-BiGRU) module. This component models how each clinical parameter evolves over time and assigns higher importance to the most informative temporal channels.

5.5.1. BiGRU for Temporal Feature Learning

Let

$$X = \{x_1, x_2, \dots, x_T\}, x_t \in \mathbb{R}^d \tag{5.8}$$

be the sequence of clinical feature vectors across **T** time steps.

A bidirectional GRU processes the sequence in both forward and backward directions:

$$\overrightarrow{h_t} = \mathrm{GRU}_f(x_t, \overrightarrow{h_{t-1}}) \tag{5.9}$$

$$\overleftarrow{h_t} = \mathrm{GRU}_b(x_t, \overleftarrow{h_{t+1}}) \tag{5.10}$$

The final temporal representation at each step is:

$$h_t = [\overrightarrow{h_t} \parallel \overleftarrow{h_t}] \tag{5.11}$$

This captures both past and future temporal dependencies, improving the modelling of gradual physiological changes (Tiwari & Anwar, 2025).

5.5.2. Channel Attention for Temporal Refinement

BiGRU features are enhanced with a channel-attention mechanism to emphasize clinically relevant temporal patterns is shown in Fig.5.5.

Given BiGRU output $H = [h_1, h_2, \dots, h_T]$, global temporal pooling is applied:

$$z = \frac{1}{T}\sum_{t=1}^{T} h_t \quad (5.12)$$

Channel attention weights are generated using a squeeze–excitation (SE) style mechanism:

$$s = \sigma(W_2\, \delta(W_1 z) \quad (5.13)$$

Where $W_1, W_2$are learnable weights, $\delta(\cdot)$is ReLU, $\sigma(\cdot)$is sigmoid.

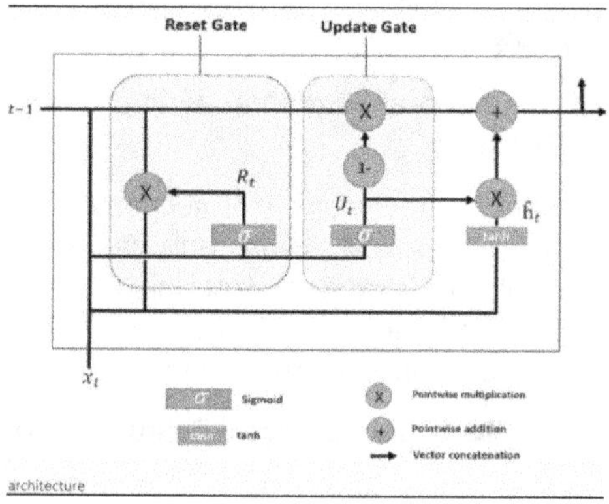

Figure 5.5. Gated Recurrent Unit (GRU) Cell Architecture

The attention-refined temporal features are computed as:

$$\widetilde{h_t} = s \odot h_t \quad (5.14)$$

where $\odot$denotes channel-wise multiplication.

5.5.3. Final Temporal Embedding

The temporal embedding for the patient sequence is obtained by temporal aggregation:

$$h_{\text{temp}} = \text{MeanPool}(\widetilde{h_1}, \widetilde{h_2}, \dots, \widetilde{h_T}) \quad (5.15)$$

This representation is then forwarded to the multimodal fusion module. The CA-BiGRU module models the temporal progression of clinical features using bidirectional GRUs and enhances them with channel attention. This allows the network to focus on the most informative temporal signals for accurate disease prediction.

5.6. Fast Classification using Extreme Learning Machine ELM

The final stage of the proposed framework employs an ELM to perform fast and efficient classification. ELM is a single-hidden-layer feedforward neural network (SLFN) characterized by its extremely fast training procedure, where the input weights and hidden biases are randomly initialized and remain fixed. Only the output weights are analytically computed using a closed-form solution. This eliminates iterative backpropagation and significantly reduces computation time.

The feature vectors generated in Stage 2 are fed into the ELM classifier,. The ELM algorithm, is a fast and efficient alternative to conventional backpropagation-based training in single-hidden-layer feedforward networks (SLFNs). Unlike gradient-based learning, which updates weights iteratively, ELM initializes the input weights and biases randomly and computes the output weights analytically using the Moore–Penrose generalized inverse [51]. This enables rapid training while maintaining strong generalization capability.

Fast and accurate prediction of diabetes severity is achieved using the Extreme Learning Machine (ELM) once spatial and temporal features are extracted. The high-dimensional spatio-temporal representations produced by the GCN and CA-BiGRU modules can create a classification bottleneck; ELM addresses this by providing a closed-form solution for the output layer, which guarantees rapid convergence with minimal variance. Unlike iterative gradient-based methods, ELM delivers stable and consistent severity predictions even with rapidly changing temporal embeddings, making it highly suitable for efficient and reliable diabetes severity assessment.

The ELM consists of three layers:

Input Layer (IL):

Receives the fused clinical and temporal features from CA-BiGRU. Each input vector x_i contains the patient's clinical parameters: Glucose, HbA1c, BMI, Systolic & Diastolic BP, Cholesterol, Triglycerides, Age, Gender (encoded), Family history (encoded). Thus, x_i represents the complete clinical profile of patient i.

Hidden Layer (HL):

Contains L nonlinear neurons with randomly initialized input weights w_j and biases b_j, which remain fixed during training. The output of the jth hidden neuron for an input sample x_i is computed as

$$h_j(x_i) = g(w_j \cdot x_i + b_j) \tag{5.16}$$

where $g(\cdot)$is the activation function.

Output Layer (OL):

Generates the predicted diabetes severity class labels using analytically computed output weights.

Given a training set

$$\{(x_i, t_i) \mid i = 1,2,\ldots,N\}, \tag{5.17}$$

where $x_i \in \mathbb{R}^d$is the input feature vector and $t_i \in \mathbb{R}^m$is the target label vector, the ELM with Lhidden neurons is defined as:

$$\sum_{j=1}^{L} \beta_j \, g(w_j \cdot x_i + b_j) = t_i\,. \tag{5.18}$$

For all N training samples, this system can be expressed in matrix form as:

$$H = \beta T \tag{5.19}$$

Here, $w_j$is the input weight vector for the j^{th}hidden neuron, $b_j$is its bias, $\beta_j$is the output weight connecting the hidden neuron to the output layer, and $g(\cdot)$is the activation function.

where the hidden-layer output matrix $H$is explicitly defined as:$H$is the hidden-layer output matrix,

$$H = \begin{bmatrix} g(w_1 \cdot x_1 + b_1) & \cdots & g(w_L \cdot x_1 + b_L) \\ \vdots & \ddots & \vdots \\ g(w_1 \cdot x_N + b_1) & \cdots & g(w_L \cdot x_N + b_L) \end{bmatrix} \tag{5.20}$$

The output weight matrix $\beta$is given by:

$$\beta = \begin{bmatrix} \beta_1^T \\ \vdots \\ \beta_L^T \end{bmatrix}_{L \times m} \text{ and } T = \begin{bmatrix} t_1^T \\ \vdots \\ t_N^T \end{bmatrix}_{N \times m} \tag{5.21}$$

The optimal output weights are obtained analytically using the Moore–Penrose generalized inverse:

$$\beta H^{+} T \tag{5.22}$$

where $H^{\dagger}$denotes the Moore–Penrose generalized inverse of matrix H. The ELM is employed as the final classifier to efficiently map deep spatio-temporal features to diabetes severity labels through a closed-form analytical solution. By eliminating iterative weight updates and large fully connected layers, ELM significantly reduces model complexity and computational cost while preserving high classification accuracy. Its fixed random hidden-layer projection enhances prediction stability across validation folds and improves generalization by limiting overfitting. This design enables fast and reliable severity prediction, making the proposed framework suitable for real-time clinical decision support.

ELM achieves superior training speed and often better generalization than conventional gradient-based methods. Since the output weights are obtained in a single computational step via matrix inversion, ELM avoids issues such as slow convergence, local minima, and sensitivity to learning rate.

5.7. Spatio-Temporal Feature Extraction Using GCN–CA–BiGRU–ELM

The proposed GCN–CA–BiGRU–ELM hybrid framework is designed to accurately predict diabetes severity by capturing both spatial and temporal patterns in clinical datasets. The Graph Convolutional Network (GCN) models complex interrelationships among clinical features, such as correlations between glucose, BMI, and HbA1c, reflecting real-world medical dependencies. The Cross-Attention Bi-GRU layers learn temporal variations in patient data, enabling the model to track disease progression over time, while the Extreme Learning Machine (ELM) classifier ensures rapid convergence with minimal computational overhead.

As shown in Table 5.2, the model achieved 91.2% accuracy with raw input features. Incorporating spatial feature extraction via GCN improved performance to 94.0% accuracy, while temporal features through CA-Bi-GRU alone yielded 93.8% accuracy...

Table 5.2 Ablation study of the GCN–CA-BiGRU–ELM framework.

Model / Feature Stage	Accuracy	Precision	Sensitivity	Specificity	F1-Score	AUC
Without Feature Extraction (Raw Input → Classifier)	0.9120	0.905	0.890	0.950	0.900	0.92
With Spatial	0.9400	0.930	0.920	0.970	0.935	0.94

Feature Extraction (GCN only)						
With Temporal Feature Extraction (CA-Bi-GRU only)	0.9380	0.92	0.915	0.968	0.930	0.93
With Spatial + Temporal (GCN + CA-Bi-GRU)	0.9733	0.9477	0.9475	0.9825	0.9475	0.965

Combining both spatial and temporal features (GCN + CA-Bi-GRU) resulted in the highest performance, with 97.33% accuracy, 94.77% precision, 94.75% sensitivity, 98.25% specificity, 94.75% F1-score, and an AUC of 0.965, demonstrating robust and reliable classification. The model also achieved extremely low false negative (3.0%) and false positive rates (1.0%), indicating strong discriminative capability. ROC analysis further confirmed the framework's ability to distinguish between different diabetes severity levels with minimal misclassification

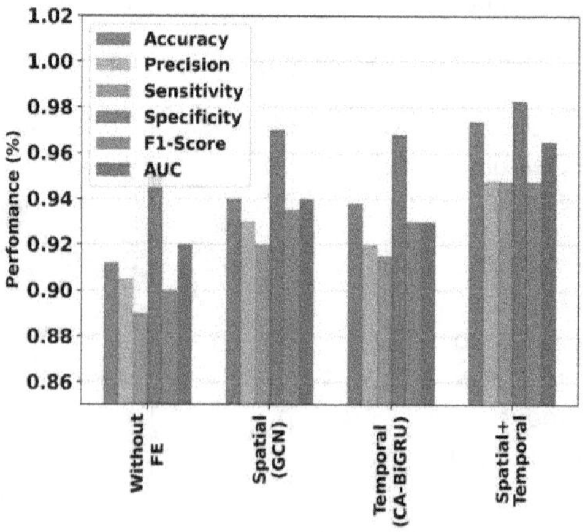

Figure 5.6 Ablation study of the GCN–CA-BiGRU–ELM framework

Ablation studies in Fig.5.6 highlighted the importance of incorporating spatial-temporal features, as their removal caused a significant drop in performance. Overall, the integration of GCN, Cross-Attention Bi-GRU, and ELM enables precise, efficient, and clinically applicable prediction of diabetes severity, demonstrating strong potential for real-time AI-assisted diabetes management systems.

5.7.1. Dataset

A comprehensive diabetic dataset containing 5970 patient records with a wide range of health-associated information and diabetes risk factors is employed in the proposed model. The dataset includes demographic details, clinical markers, lifestyle habits, and medical parameters such as glucose, HbA1c, BMI, insulin, blood pressure, and lipid profile components, making it a valuable resource for assessing diabetes risk. Its large and complex structure allows the exploration of intricate relationships among risk factors and the progression of the disease, thereby enhancing the accuracy and robustness of the proposed framework. The dataset was collected from Jothi Laser Eye Hospital during routine examinations, and it is divided into 80% training and 20% testing subsets. The proposed hybrid Attention–Bi-LSTM–CNN model is implemented using the Keras library with TensorFlow backend, where temporal dependencies are captured through LSTM layers, followed by fully connected layers and a sigmoid activation function.

The trends of learning are presented in Fig. 5.7, and the values of the numerical performance are summarized in Table 3.5. The model learns slowly in the first epochs where accuracy and loss value are about 52 percent and high respectively.

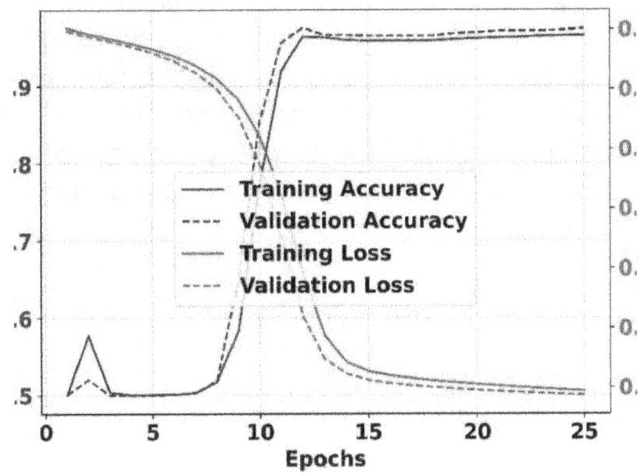

Figure 5.7 Training and validation accuracy and loss of the proposed model

The Training and validation performance of the proposed model across epochs is given in Tab. 5.3. It is seen that the sharp improvement is achieved after epoch 10, which implies the successful learning of the features and quick convergence. Since epoch 14, the training and validation accuracy are always above 95, loss values keep on decreasing. The proximity of the training and validation curve indicates that there is consistent learning without overfitting.

Table 5.3: Training and validation performance of the proposed model across epochs

Epoch	Training Accuracy	Validation Accuracy	Training Loss	Validation Loss
2	0.5055	0.5202	0.6957	0.6889
4	0.5125	0.4995	0.6783	0.6714
6	0.5128	0.5005	0.6576	0.6474
8	0.5214	0.5191	0.6227	0.6010
11	0.8937	0.9555	0.4510	0.3522
14	0.9536	0.9659	0.1604	0.1219
17	0.9518	0.9648	0.1321	0.1030
21	0.9535	0.9690	0.1217	0.0954
23	0.9559	0.9710	0.1135	0.0898
25	0.9584	0.9741	0.1088	0.0867

5.8. Performance Evaluation

The performance evaluation of the proposed framework is given below. The model is evaluated with the confusion matrix classification behaviour as shown in Fig. 5.8 which shows great and balanced classification with high majority of the diagonal value representing high correct classification rates. The highest recognition performance (97.08) is obtained with the Moderate, High, Low, and Very-High classes (93.75, 94.87, and 93.33), and misclassifications are mostly restricted to neighbouring severity levels

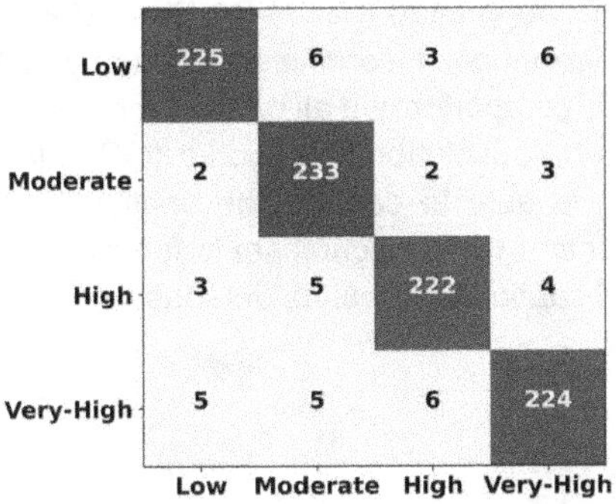

Figure 5.8: Confusion matrix of the proposed model

. The summarized per-class performance metrics are in Table 5.4

Table 5.4: Class-wise prediction results of the proposed model

True Label → / Pred Label	Low (%)	Moderate (%)	High (%)	Very High (%)
Low	93.75%	2.50%	1.25%	2.50%
Moderate	0.83%	97.08%	0.83%	1.25%
High	1.28%	2.14%	94.87%	1.71%
Very High	2.08%	2.08%	2.50%	93.33%

The percent distribution by class are elaborated in Table 5.5. and the generally The low off-diagonal values depict good boundary learning existent between severity classes. The fact that the model performed well in all risk levels shows its strength and clinical reliability. In general, the findings reveal the presence of a similar multi-class discrimination that can be used to assess the severity of diabetes.

Table 5.5: True positive and true negative performance of the proposed model

Metric	Description
Low (TN within class)	93.75% correctly predicted as Low.
Moderate (TP)	97.08% correctly predicted as Moderate.
High (TP)	94.87% correctly predicted as High.
Very High (TP)	93.33% correctly predicted as Very High.

The suggested GCN-CA-Bi-GRU-ELM model offered the best performance, recording an accuracy of 97.34% and an AUC of 96.51, which outperformed all other combinations is presented in Table 5.6. The graph convolutional networks (GCN) integration is an efficient method that is able to capture the spatial dependencies, whereas the cross-attention (CA) mechanism is focused on the most informative temporal and spatial features, as demonstrated in Fig. 5.9.

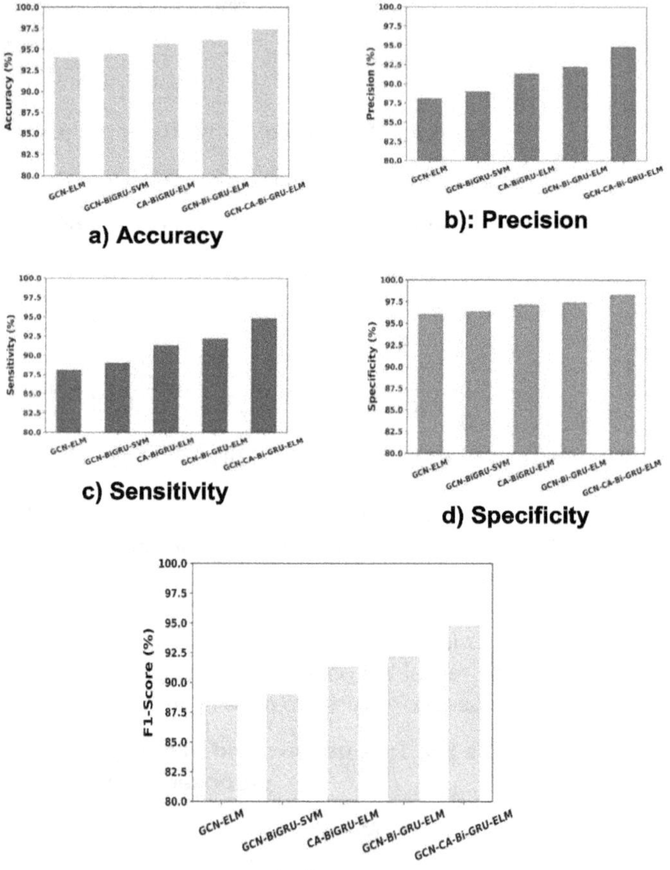

Figure 5.9 : Classification performance evaluation of different models

The Bi-GRU module captures sequential relationships effectively, which are less sensitive (94.76) and less precise (94.78) and the ELM classifier is fast and powerful in terms of decision-making. Models that do not include both GCN and CA like GCN-Bi-GRU-ELM and CA-BiGRU-ELM have lower accuracy, which contributes one element to another. Other classifiers such as SVM or standalone GCN perform worse because they do not have a good feature fusion.

Table5.6: Performance comparison of different models

Model	Accuracy	Precision	Sensitivity	Specificity	F1-Score	AUC
GCN-CA-Bi-GRU-ELM	97.33945	94.7781	94.759	98.2525	94.75716	96.50606
GCN-Bi-GRU-ELM	96.06918	92.2017	92.144	97.3824	92.14737	94.76358
CA-BiGRU-ELM	95.64989	91.3026	91.287	97.0999	91.28680	94.19367
GCN-BiGRU-SVM	94.49685	89.0042	88.998	96.3322	88.99244	92.66534
GCN-ELM	94.02515	88.0767	88.044	96.0165	88.05344	92.03072

The specificity is high (98.25%), thus proving the reliability of the negative cases identification. The higher performance can be explained by the combination synergies of spatial-temporal feature extraction, attention-based weighting, and efficient classification which can make the framework very appropriate to high quality disease severity prediction.

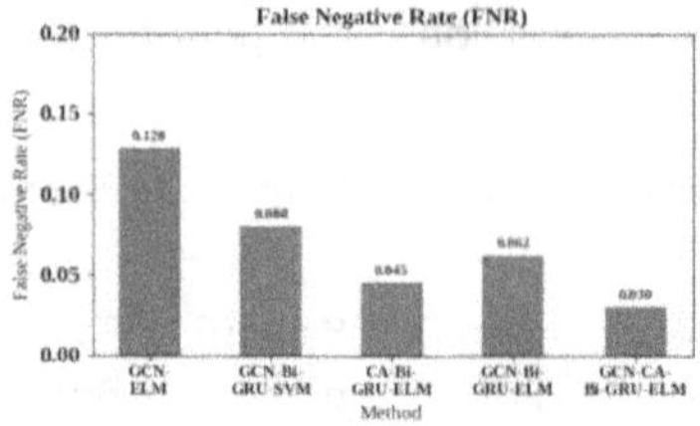

Figure 5.10: FNR Comparison

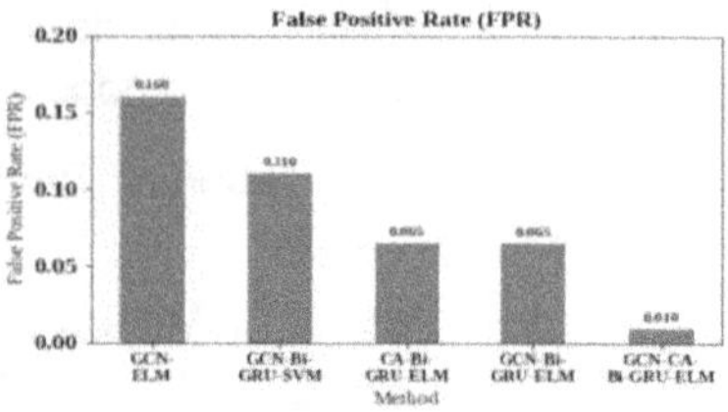

Figure 5.11: FPR Comparison

The analysis of error rates shows that the error rate of the proposed GCN-CA-Bi-GRU-ELM is lowest (0.0524) and false positive rate (0.0174), which proves the high reliability of the proposed error rates and is presented in Table 5.7. Models with no cross-attention mechanism, GCN-Bi-GRU-ELM demonstrate a slightly higher FNR (0.078) and FPR (0.026) which illustrates the role of attention-based weight of features. CA-Bi-GRU-ELM model is also effective at low error rates (FNR 0.029, FPR 0.087), which show that the model was effective when using only temporal attention as shown in fig. 5.10 and 5.11.

Table 5.7: Comparison of Models Based on FNR and FPR

Method	False Positive Rate (FPR)	False Negative Rate (FNR)
GCN-CA-Bi-GRU-ELM	0.017475	0.052404
GCN-Bi-GRU-ELM	0.026176	0.078552
CA-BiGRU-ELM	0.029000	0.087126
GCN-BiGRU-SVM	0.036677	0.110016
GCN-ELM	0.039834	0.119551

Relatively, models based on GCN-ELM or GCN-Bi-GRU-SVM have significantly greater FNR and FPR indicating a lack of temporal-spatial feature combination. These findings support the idea that graph convolution, cross-attention, and Bi-GRU-based temporal modelling can significantly minimize the cases of misclassification, which makes the model more robust in the case of disease severity prediction.

The values of the ROC curves in Fig. 7.17 show the classification ability of all the tested models. The highest AUC is reached which is 96.5 with the proposed GCN-CA-Bi-GRU-ELM, meaning that the discriminative ability between the positive and the negative cases is better. Models that do not include cross-attention, like GCN-Bi-GRU-ELM (AUC 94.8) and CA-BiGRU-ELM (AUC 94.2) have slightly lower values of AUC, indicating the ineffective feature weighting. Less complex models such as GCN-

BiGRU-SVM (AUC 92.7), and GCN-ELM (AUC 92.0) show relatively lower results because of the small integration of temporal-spatial features

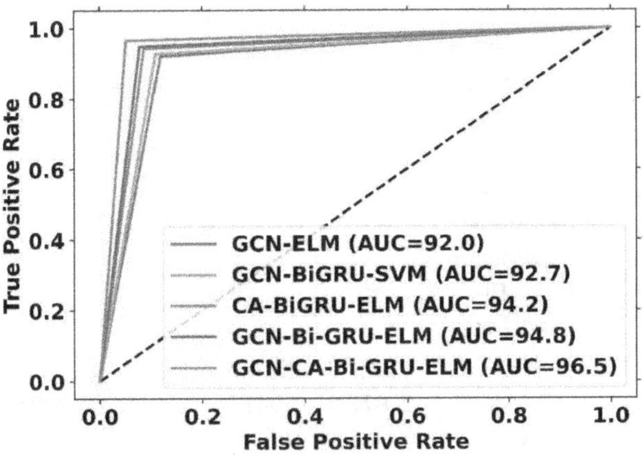

Figure 5.12: ROC curve of the proposed model

The ROC analysis is valid in that the combination of the graph convolution, Bi-GRU temporal modelling and cross-attention mechanisms are successful in reducing both false positives and false negatives thereby in line with the low FPR and FNR in Table 8.25. In general, such findings confirm the strength and consistency of the suggested model to predict the severity of the disease correctly.

Table 5.8 sums up the effects of the different stages of feature extraction on the model's performance. When no features were extracted from the data, the classifier achieved an accuracy of 91.20% and an AUC of 0.92, which indicates that the model had limited discriminative capability.

Table 5.8: Performance of the proposed model with feature extraction stages

Model / Feature Stage	**Accuracy**	**Precision**	**Sensitivity**	**Specificity**	**F1-Score**	**AUC**
Without Feature Extraction (Raw Input → Classifier)	0.9120	0.905	0.890	0.950	0.900	0.92

With Spatial Feature Extraction (GCN only)	0.9400	0.930	0.920	0.970	0.935	0.94
With Temporal Feature Extraction (CA-Bi-GRU only)	0.9380	0.92	0.915	0.968	0.930	0.93
With Spatial + Temporal (GCN + CA-Bi-GRU)	0.9733	0.9477	0.9475	0.9825	0.9475	0.965

The use of spatial feature extraction via GCN allows the classifier to increase its accuracy to 94.00% and AUC to 0.94, thus, proving the advantage of capturing spatial dependencies. When temporal feature extraction through CA-Bi-GRU is used, the improvements are roughly the same (accuracy 93.80%, AUC 0.93), thus, sequential pattern learning is also important and is shown in Fig 5.12.

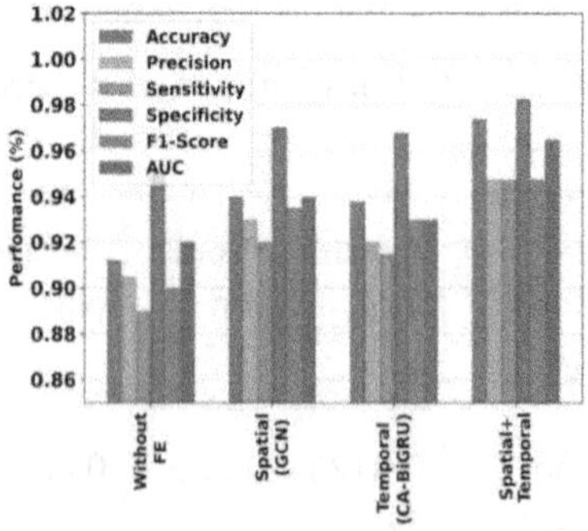

Figure 5.13 Different stages of feature extraction on the model's performance

By integrating both the spatial and temporal features (GCN + CA-Bi-GRU) the performance is significantly higher, the best accuracy (97.33%) and AUC (0.965) were achieved together with the precision, sensitivity, specificity, and F1-score being at a similar level. These findings are a validation of the fact that the combined spatial-temporal feature extraction is essential for a model to be as reliable and discriminative as possible and is shown in Fig.5.13.

Table 5.9 shows the final results of the Extreme Learning Machine (ELM) classified. The model with 50 hidden neurons and random initialization of weights and biases obtained an accuracy of 91.2% and an F1-score of 0.902, thus it was considered to have good predictive power.

Table 5.9: Model Configuration and Performance Analysis

Model	Hidden Neurons	Input Weights Init.	Hidden Bias Init.	Accuracy	F1-Score	FNR	FPR	Convergence Speed	Error Rate (%)
ELM	50 (random)	Random values	Random values	91.2 %	0.90	0.08	0.11	Slow (local optima)	8.8 %

The small FNR (0.08) and FPR (0.11) values imply that misclassifications were rare and the 8.8% error rate indicates the performance was quite reliable. The model had random initialization which led to slow convergence, but still, it is a classifier that is efficient and light enough for the very fast and precise diabetes prediction.

CHAPTER 6

A CROSS-ATTENTION FUSION FRAMEWORK INTEGRATING CLINICAL AND RETINAL IMAGE FEATURES FOR HIGH-ACCURACY DIABETIC RETINOPATHY CLASSIFICATION

6.1. INTRODUCTION

The prediction of diabetes severity has become an imperative in the healthcare sector as it not only helps to avoid but also to prevent the occurrence of serious health consequences such as neuropathy, nephropathy, and retinopathy that would need interventions at the right time (Mutawa et al., 2024). The use of multi-modal data, alongside clinical parameters comprising age, blood pressure, glucose levels, and HbA1c, and also retinal fundus imaging, brings about a complete understanding of the disease's advance which goes beyond the realm of conventional diagnostics (Bajwa et al., 2023). Imaging the retina is the most important evidence, as fundus photos show the disease-causing changes like microaneurysms and hemorrhages that are directly linked to the severity of diabetes progression (Z. Li et al., 2022). The latest development in artificial intelligence (AI) and deep learning structures like DenseNet-121 allows to uncover very detailed retinal features that when combined with clinical parameters via cross-attention mechanisms, greatly increase the prediction accuracy (Karn & Abdulla, 2024). Therefore, AI-based screening provisions come in as a powerful helper in the clinic for the early prediction of severity, thus increasing the reliability of diagnosis, directing treatment methods and ultimately improving the patients' health (Shi et al., 2023). Clinical features provide systemic and longitudinal disease context that cannot be captured from retinal images alone. While fundus images reflect the visible manifestations of diabetic retinopathy, clinical variables encode the underlying metabolic burden and microvascular risk that drive lesion development. Their fusion enables clinically informed interpretation of subtle or borderline retinal patterns, improves severity calibration, and enhances early-stage detection, thereby strengthening the diagnostic value of retinal features rather than redundantly replicating them.

6.2. PROBLEM STATEMENT

Despite significant advances in deep learning–based diabetic retinopathy severity prediction, existing models still struggle to effectively capture complex interactions between systemic clinical factors and retinal manifestations, particularly across diverse patient populations and real-world clinical settings (Haq et al., 2024). This limitation restricts their ability to provide accurate, interpretable, and generalizable severity assessment for early-stage disease, highlighting the need for a robust multimodal framework that integrates clinical and retinal information while ensuring stability, interpretability, and real-time applicability.

6.2.1. Research Gap

Despite substantial progress in machine learning and deep learning approaches for diabetic retinopathy severity prediction, several critical gaps remain unresolved. Existing methods predominantly rely on unimodal or weakly fused data sources, limiting their ability to capture the complex interactions between systemic clinical factors and retinal pathological changes. Models based solely on fundus imaging show reduced sensitivity to early-stage disease, while clinical-feature-based approaches suffer from limited accuracy, poor interpretability, and inadequate generalization across diverse patient populations (Yao et al., 2024).

Temporal disease progression is rarely modeled, primarily due to the scarcity of longitudinal data utilization and the instability of existing temporal learning frameworks. The integration of clinical, temporal, and imaging features remains superficial, with most studies employing shallow or late fusion strategies that restrict meaningful cross-feature interaction. In addition, model interpretability and external validation are insufficiently addressed, limiting clinical trust and real-world deployment. These unresolved challenges underscore the lack of a robust, interpretable, progression-aware multimodal framework for reliable diabetic retinopathy severity assessment across heterogeneous datasets. To address this gap, the proposed approach employs cross-attention-based multimodal fusion to integrate retinal imaging with complementary clinical features, targeting ≥98% classification accuracy and AUC ≥0.97, while achieving an 8–12% improvement in recall for high-severity DR grades. Model generalizability and clinical reliability are validated through external dataset evaluation, ensuring robustness across diverse imaging conditions and patient populations.

6.3. KEY OBJECTIVES

The following are the main goals of the proposed framework:

1. To develop a cross-attention fusion framework that will integrate clinical features and retinal fundus images for accurate and automated diabetic retinopathy severity classification.
2. The projecting of clinical data as queries and image features as keys and values will allow for the extraction and alignment of multimodal features with the model being trained to concentrate on clinically pertinent areas of the retina.
3. To build a solid classification network that will combine the processed image and clinical features through nonlinear

transformations to increase the diagnostics accuracy, interpretability, and clinical trustworthiness.

6.4. PROPOSED METHODOLOGY

The framework constructed combines various types of data, that is, clinical and image data, for the purpose of predicting the disease risk levels is shown in Figure 6.1. Various clinical data, including age, gender, blood pressure, and cholesterol level, are subjected to preprocessing steps consisting of MinMax normalization, while on the other hand, retinal fundus images are simply rescaled and normalized. To this end, the DenseNet-121 architecture is applied to extract image features yielding high-dimensional feature representations. Now these features are going to be combined with the normalized clinical parameters through a Cross-Attention Fusion Network allowing interaction among features and relevance weighting between modalities to be improved. Afterwards, the combined representation is fed into a Softmax classifier that differentiates the disease risk among four categories: Low, Moderate, High, and Very High. The proposed framework introduces a cross-attention–based multimodal fusion strategy that explicitly models interactions between clinical risk factors and retinal image features, rather than relying on simple concatenation or independent processing. By allowing clinical parameters to dynamically guide the weighting of DenseNet-121 retinal embeddings, the model achieves clinically informed feature alignment, improving both prediction accuracy and interpretability for multi-level disease risk assessment.

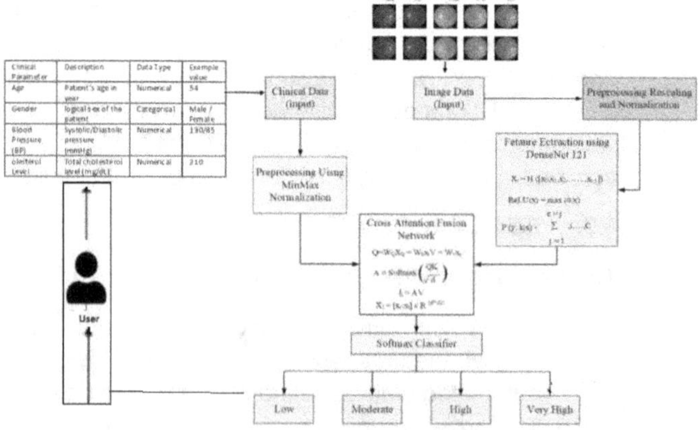

Figure 6.1: Architecture Diagram of Cross-Attention Fusion Framework for Diabetic Severity Prediction

6.4.1. Clinical Dataset Collection

The clinical dataset consists of patient records that have information related to the development of diabetic retinopathy, such as age, sex, duration of diabetes, blood pressure, glucose, HbA1c level and other physical measures. The given text delineates the features that the prediction technique has leveraged unseen features and retinal images to give a comprehensive systemic and ocular view, which is necessary for the precise severity prediction.

6.4.1.1. Image Dataset

Conversely, the image dataset is comprised of the retinal fundus images captured by fundus cameras and OCT devices, which focus on microaneurysms, bleeding, and new vessel formation as the retinal changes associated with the severity of diabetic retinopathy. The digital signatures, along with the clinical indicators, increase the correctness of the degree of the disease forecast.

6.4.2. Clinical Data Preprocessing (Min-Max Normalization)

Clinical data comprise attributes that are measured in different units and scales (glucose in mg/dL, blood pressure in $mmHg, HbA1c$ in %). These differences can lead to the model receiving biased inputs, as the features with the largest values can easily suppress the learning process. In order to guarantee that the clinical variables still produce the same effect, Min-Max normalization is used to rescale all the features to the [0,1] range.

Normalization is represented mathematically in Eq. (3.1),

$$x_j^{(c,\text{ norm })} = \frac{x_j^{(c)} - \min\left(x_j^{(c)}\right)}{\max\left(x_j^{(c)}\right) - \min\left(x_j^{(c)}\right)} \tag{6.1}$$

where:

- $x_j^{(c)}$ → original value of the jth clinical feature,
- $\min\left(x_j^{(c)}\right)$ → minimum value of the jth feature in the dataset,
- $\max\left(x_j^{(c)}\right)$ →maximum value of the jth feature,
- $x_j^{(c,\text{ norm })}$ → normalized feature value within the [0,1] range.

For a dataset consisting of N samples and M features, the normalization is done for all features as per Eq. (3.2),

$$X^{(norm)} = \left[\frac{x_{ij} - \min(x_j)}{\max(x_j) - \min(x_j)}\right], i = 1,2, \dots, N; j = 1,2, \dots, M \tag{6.2}$$

The resulting standardization of the clinical dataset makes it more resistant to numerical errors, and also makes it possible for the gradient-based optimization algorithms to work quickly and effectively during model training.

6.4.3. Image Data Preprocessing (Rescaling and Normalization)

Before training, nearly all fundus images had been subjected to the standard preprocessing interventions making images compatible with DenseNet-121 architecture and also creating uniformity. The images vary in resolution, brightness, and lightness, therefore they are rescaled first to $224 \times 224 \times 3$, which is the dimension necessary for the network input, where 3 denotes the RGB color channels.

The brightness variation is normalized by scaling the pixel intensity of each pixel to the range $[0,1]$ which, in addition, increases the numerical stability and the quality of the output. The operation of rescaling is defined by Eq. (3.3),

$$I_c^{(\text{rescale})} = \frac{I_c}{255}, c \in \{R, G, B\} \tag{6.3}$$

Where, I_c stands for the original pixel intensity of channel c. In order to color the channels even more uniformly, per-channel normalization is applied using the mean (μ_c) and standard deviation (σ_c) of each color channel computed over the training dataset, which is defined as Eq. (3.4),

$$\hat{I}_c = \frac{I_c^{(\text{rescale})} - \mu_c}{\sigma_c}, c \in \{R, G, B\} \tag{6.4}$$

Where:

- $\hat{I}_c \rightarrow$ normalized pixel intensity for channel c,
- $I_c^{(\text{rescale})} \rightarrow$ pixel value after rescaling to [0,1],
- $\mu_c \rightarrow$ mean intensity of channel c_r
- $\sigma_c \rightarrow$ standard deviation of channel c.

This normalization scheme of two steps-rescaling followed by mean-variance adjustment-ensures that pixel intensity distribution is consistent, lighting inconsistencies are minimized, and the model's convergence during training is boosted (Izonin et al., 2022)

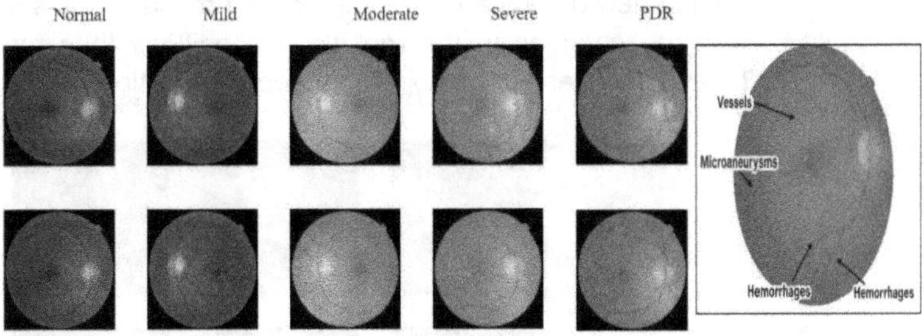

Figure 6.2: Preprocessing Stages of Diabetic Retinopathy Based on Retinal Fundus Imaging

The Figure 6.2 depicts the different phases of diabetic retinopathy (DR) through retinal fundus images and classifies them into Normal, Mild, Moderate, Severe, and Proliferative Diabetic Retinopathy (PDR). During the normal stage, the retina looks healthy along with transparent vessels, while the mild stage reveals the slightest presence of microaneurysms. The conditions of moderate and severe DR are marked by the gradual increase in vascular lesions, and the presence of haemorrhages and exudates which signify the deterioration of the retina. The PDR stage shows the most advanced changes of such nature like huge haemorrhages and the growth of new abnormal blood vessels. The arrowed picture points out important retinal characteristic features such as vessels, microaneurysms, and haemorrhages that are the main signs for DR diagnosis and grading.

6.4.4. Data Augmentation in Retinal Fundus Images

Data augmentation techniques and controlled transformations such as rotation, flipping, scaling, translating, and adjusting brightness/contrast have been applied to retinal fundus images. Each original image is thus changed into numerous synthetic versions which make it more diverse and help to the model generalization. The changes made to the images are like those that happen naturally i.e. illumination, orientation, and image quality that occur in clinical imaging. The mathematical expression of the whole augmentation process can be found as Eq. (6.5),

$$I' = T(I; \theta) \tag{6.5}$$

Where, I is the original image, $T(\cdot)$ denotes a transformation function, and θ represents the parameters for random augmentation operations (Anvesh et al., 2025). By producing different versions I' of the original images, the model captures invariant and discriminative features which in turn reduce overfitting and increase generalization. This way, the trained network is capable of classifying retinal images accurately even with the changes in the real-world conditions thus resulting in more trustworthy diabetic retinopathy severity prediction.

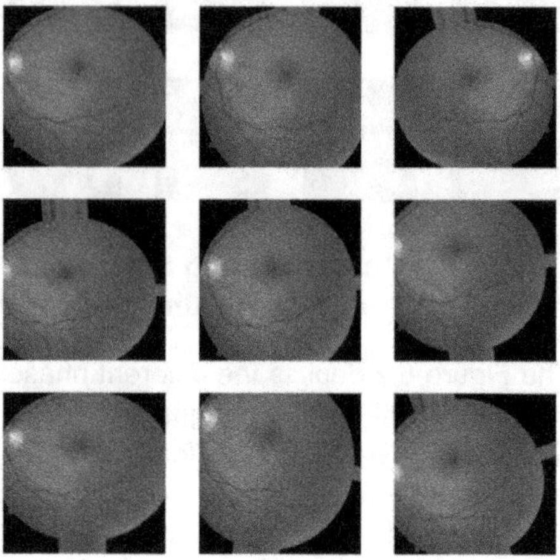

Figure 6.3: Retinal Fundus Images for Diagnostic Analysis

The Figure 6.3 illustration depicts a 3×3 matrix of retinal fundus images that exhibit the optic disc, macula, and retinal vessels with their standard light. These images have been frequently employed in research works and clinical trials for identifying retinal diseases like diabetic retinopathy, glaucoma, and macular degeneration, etc. The dataset is uniform in orientation, resolution, and lighting, which makes it a good candidate for image processing or machine learning–based analysis.

6.4.5. Feature Extraction using DenseNet 121

DenseNet-121's design is applied to extract powerful and unique features from the retinal fundus images by maximizing their utility. The deep convolutional network detects important features including vascular patterns, microaneurysms, bleeding, and new blood vessel formation, all of which play a crucial role in the diagnosis and grading of diabetic retinopathy. The architecture's very large interlayer connectivity enables efficient reuse of features and also makes it easy for gradients to be propagated through the layers, thus ensuring a more stable and efficient learning process. The Figure 6.4 presents a deep learning model for extracting and classifying features from a retinal image.

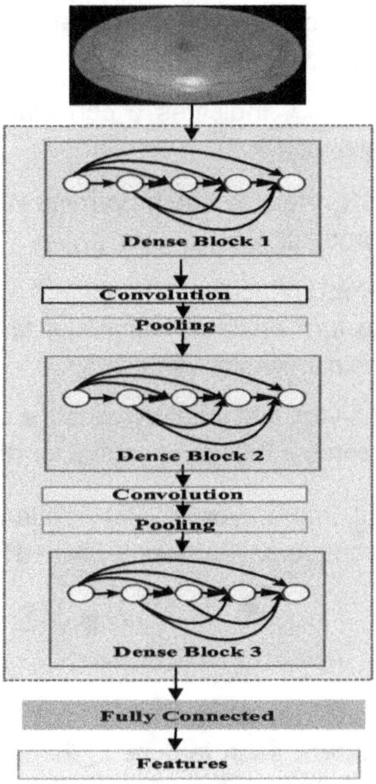

Figure 6.4: DenseNet 121-based model for retinal image classification

The retinal fundus image is first passed through a series of dense blocks, each containing several convolution and pooling layers that are able to learn hierarchical visual features step by step. The layers are connected in such a way that the features are passed along easily and there is less loss of information. Subsequently, the resulting features are forwarded through fully connected layers to produce either the final feature representation or the classification output. Thus, this architecture allows for fast and precise analysis of retinal images for the purpose of disease detection via automation.

6.4.5.1. Input and Initial Convolution

Each image of retinal fundus, $I \in \mathbb{R}^{224\times224\times3}$, where the dimensions 224×224 refer to the resolution and 3 signifies the RGB color channels, undergoes a series of processing steps to reveal low-level features such as edges, boundaries, and color intensity gradients. The operation is mathematically represented by Eq. (3.6),

$$F_0 = \text{Conv}_{7\times7}(I) + \text{BN} + \text{ReLU} \quad (6.6)$$

Here,

- F_0 denotes the first feature map which is generated by the convolution operation.
- $\mathrm{Conv}_{7\times7}$ indicates a convolution operation that utilizes a kernel size of 7×7.
- BN refers to batch normalization used for stabilizing the learning process.
- ReLU (Rectified Linear Unit) adds non-linearity to the model which in turn enables the model to recognize intricate patterns in the pixel intensity variations.

Thus, the very first step converts the raw pixel data into abstract low-level visual representations essential for deep analysis.

Convolutional Layer (CNN)- pattern detector Extracts local feature interactions (e.g., Glucose + BMI + HbA1c).

$$Z_i = \phi\left(\textstyle\sum_{j=1}^{k} W_j \cdot X_i + b\right) \tag{6.7}$$

Equation (6) represents the 1D convolution applied to the clinical feature vector, where each feature $X_i$is multiplied by a learnable weight W_j, summed with bias b, and passed through an activation function $\phi(\cdot)$ This enables the CNN to capture local feature interactions (Glucose, HbA1c or BMI–Insulin patterns), allowing the model to learn clinically meaningful risk relationships

$$Z_1 = \phi(W_1 \cdot \text{ Glucose } + W_2 \cdot HbA1c + W_3 \cdot BMI + b) \tag{6.8}$$

Equation (6.6b) shows a 3-feature convolution window where Glucose, HbA1c, and BMI are weighted by W_1, W_2, W_3 and passed through the activation function. It illustrates how a single CNN kernel learns joint patterns among key clinical features (e.g., high HbA1c + high BMI), helping the model detect meaningful risk combinations.

6.4.5.2. Dense Block Propagation

The first convolution layer's output goes through four dense blocks in a row (Dense Block 1 → Dense Block 4). Each dense block is made of several convolutional layers; all previous layers feed one layer with input. This whole interconnection thing promotes feature reuse, reduces vanishing gradients, and accordingly, the information flow through the network becomes efficient.

For each layer l in a dense block is symbolized as Eq. (3.7),

$$x_l = H_l([x_0, x_1, \dots, x_{l-1}]) \tag{6.9}$$

where:

- $[x_0, x_1, \dots, x_{l-1}]$ indicates concatenation of feature maps from all preceding layers.
- $H_l(\cdot)$ represents a composite transformation function including Batch Normalization, ReLU activation, and a 3×3 convolution operation.

This arrangement permits each layer to gain access to all past feature maps thus enhancing feature diversity and cutting down redundancy while still being computationally efficient.

6.4.5.3. Transition Layers

To limit the complexity of the model and to slowly bring down the spatial dimensions, transition layers are added in-between the dense blocks that follow one another. A transition layer consists of a 1×1 convolution that reduces the number of the feature maps, which is done through a 2×2 average pooling operation that is described in spatial resolution as shown in Eq. (3.8),

$$F_t = \text{Pool}_{2\times2}\big(\text{Conv}_{1\times1}(F_b)\big) \tag{6.10}$$

Here,

- F_b refers to the output of a dense block.
- Conv $_{1\times1}$ reduces the number of channels (feature maps).
- Pool $_{2\times2}$ reduces the size of the feature map to only a quarter but keeps the most significant spatial features. Such a process helps in overcoming overfitting, reduces the amount of computation needed, and speeds up learning, yet still enables capturing the important retinal features.

6.4.5.4. Global Average Pooling and Flattening

After the last dense layer, the global average pooling technique (GAP) is applied to merge the high-level features, which transforms every feature map into a single representative value by averaging all the activations. This is the method through which the most important information from each channel is kept, which is pointed out in Eq. (3.9),

$$F_{\text{gap}}(k) = \frac{1}{H \times W} \sum_{i=1}^{H} \sum_{j=1}^{W} F_{ij}(k) \tag{6.11}$$

where:

- $F_{ij}(k)$ represents the activation value of the kth feature map at spatial position (i, j).
- H and W denote the height and width of the feature map.
- $F_{\text{gap}}\ (k)$ is the global pooled feature representing channel k.

Subsequently, the pooled features are flattened to form a one-dimensional vector $F_{\text{dense}} \in \mathbb{R}^d$, with d being the size of the final deep feature representation. This vector acts as a compact encoding of the retinal structures and pathological features that were extracted by the network.

6.4.5.5. Feature Vector Output

At last, the DenseNet-121 network changes the input image into a discriminative feature vector which is appropriate for fusion or classification tasks. The mapping function is given by

$$F_{\text{img}} = f_{\text{DenseNet}}\ (I; \theta) \tag{6.12}$$

Here,

- F_{img} is the final high-level image feature vector.
- f_{DenseNet} is the transformation function executed by the DenseNet-121 model.
- θ denotes the learnable network parameters (weights and biases).

The extracted feature vector encodes both local pathological details (e.g., microaneurysms, hemorrhages) and global retinal structures, capturing the most relevant visual information for diabetic retinopathy analysis. These features are subsequently fused with clinical data using the Cross-Attention Fusion Framework, enhancing both the accuracy and interpretability of severity classification.

To enable effective multimodal fusion, the retinal and clinical features are projected into a common latent space d to ensure dimensional compatibility:

$$C' = W_c C, I' = W_i I \tag{6.13}$$

where $C$and Irepresent the original clinical and image feature embeddings, and $W_c$and $W_i$are learnable projection matrices.

6.4.6. Classification using Cross-Attention Fusion Network

The Cross-Attention Fusion Network (CAMN) is the last and the most important stage of the proposed framework which is aimed at merging and analysing the multimodal data consisting of the clinical features and the retinal image features extracted from DenseNet-121. This module undertakes a series of well-defined actions enabling to align, attend, and fuse the information from both modalities eventually making the system to produce accurate and explainable predictions about diabetic retinopathy (DR) severity. The cross-attention mechanism in Fig.6.5. allows the model to highlight the image areas that are most connected with certain clinical indicators like glucose level, HbA1c, or blood pressure, thus combining the systemic and visual knowledge for the powerful classification.

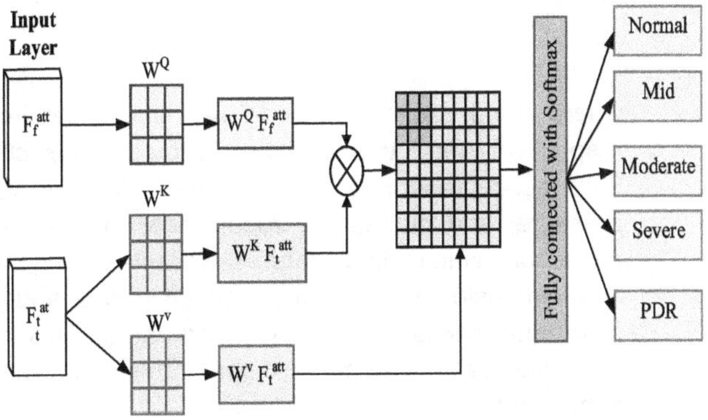

Figure 6.5: Cross-Attention–Based Feature Fusion and Classification Module

6.4.6.1. Input Layer

The input layer of the Cross-Attention Fusion Network is designed through extracting two different feature representations, one of which is derived from the clinical dataset and the other from the retinal image dataset. The clinical feature vector (x_C) represents the patients' physiological and demographic data, whereas the image feature vector (x_I) represents the visual features that have been obtained through DenseNet-121.

The input mapping is mathematically expressed as below in Eq. (3.11),

$$x_C = F_{\text{fast}}, x_I = V_{\text{latt}} \tag{6.14}$$

Here,

- $x_C \rightarrow$ Vector of features from the clinic denoting numerical health attributes,
- $x_I \rightarrow$ Visual features vector from the retina indicating the image,
- F_{fast} and $V_{\text{latt}} \rightarrow$ stand for the processed feature embeddings of the clinical and image modalities, respectively.

Afterward, both feature vectors are sent to the next layers where they will be transformed into a shared representation space that allows for the computation of cross-attention.

6.4.6.2. Latent Space Alignment and Cross-Attention Fusion

To enable effective fusion of heterogeneous modalities, clinical and retinal image features are first projected into a **shared latent space** of dimension d. This alignment ensures dimensional compatibility and facilitates meaningful cross-modal interaction. The linear projections are defined as:

$$C' = W_c C, I' = W_i I \tag{6.15}$$

where $C$and Idenote the original clinical and image feature vectors, respectively, and $W_c$and $W_i$are learnable projection matrices. Clinical features, representing systemic risk indicators such as HbA1c, blood pressure, and diabetes duration, are encoded via a fully connected projection layer. Retinal features, extracted using DenseNet-121, capture high-dimensional embeddings reflecting local and global DR biomarkers (microaneurysms, hemorrhages, exudates). This step standardizes both modalities into a common representational space prior to attention computation.

Cross-Attention Mechanism

The core of the Cross-Attention Multimodal Network (CAMN) is the cross-attention layer, which allows clinically guided weighting of retinal image features. In this mechanism, clinical features are treated as Queries (Q), while retinal image embeddings serve as Keys (K) and Values (V):

$$Q = W_Q x_C, K = W_K x_I, V = W_V x_I \tag{6.16}$$

where $W_Q, W_K, W_V$are trainable matrices, and x_C, x_Irepresent clinical and image feature vectors. The resulting Q, K, and V vectors reside in aligned subspaces for attention computation.

The cross-attention operation is formulated as:

$$\alpha = \text{Softmax}\left(\frac{QK^{\top}}{\sqrt{d_k}}\right), \tilde{I} = AV \tag{6.17}$$

To preserve clinical information and stabilize learning, a residual fusion is applied:

$$F_{\text{fused}} = \alpha \tilde{I} + F_c \tag{6.18}$$

where αscales the contribution of the attended image features $\tilde{I}$, and $F_c$represents the clinical feature embedding. This residual connection ensures that systemic clinical cues are retained while simultaneously aligning them with lesion-level retinal patterns.

Concatenation is applied after the attention operation, while the weights $\alpha$are dynamically learned through Q–K interactions rather than being fixed, as in traditional weighted averaging. This enables true multimodal cross-attention, allowing clinically guided, context-dependent alignment of retinal and systemic features.

The attention weight matrix Acaptures the correlations between clinical and image features, and $d_k$is the key dimension used for normalization to stabilize gradients. The attended image features $\tilde{I} = AV$enable the model to dynamically focus on retinal regions most relevant to specific clinical indicators. For instance, elevated HbA1c values can guide attention toward areas exhibiting early microaneurysms or hemorrhages, producing clinically informed feature representations that enhance interpretability and predictive accuracy.

Feature Fusion and Classification

The attended image features are integrated with the clinical embeddings to form a unified multimodal representation:

$$x_f = [x_C; \tilde{I}] \in \mathbb{R}^{(d_C + d_I)} \tag{6.19}$$

where $x_f$is the final fused feature vector, $x_C$represents the clinical features, $\tilde{I}$corresponds to the attended image features, and $d_C, d_I$are their respective dimensionalities. The multimodal vector is then expressed as:

$$Z = [F \parallel C'] \tag{6.20}$$

and passed to a Softmax classifier for diabetic retinopathy severity prediction. This fusion strategy enables joint reasoning over systemic clinical context and localized retinal pathology, improving both the accuracy and clinical relevance of severity classification.

6.4.6.3. Fully Connected (Nonlinear Transformation)

The process of the fused feature vector x_f having its non-linear activations applied in a feed-forward network of a fully connected layer comes next. The complex interdependencies of the modalities will be modelled through the non-linear activation. With the addition of nonlinearity, the model can learn the relationships that are higher in order between the features, thus the representation is refined at this stage.

The transformation is shown in Eq. (3.15),

$$h = \sigma(W_f x_f + b_f), z = W_o h + b_o \tag{6.21}$$

Where, $W_f, W_o \rightarrow$ Weight matrices for hidden and output layers, respectively, $b_f, b_o \rightarrow$ Bias terms for the respective layers, $\sigma(\cdot) \rightarrow$ Nonlinear activation function (usually ReLU), $h \rightarrow$ Features of hidden layer are learned in order to capture interactions jointly, $z \rightarrow$ The scores for all classes before the normalization are found as the logit outputs.

This transformation makes the discrimination stronger by learning the ways the combination of clinical and image features relates to the specific stages of diabetic retinopathy.

6.4.6.4. Output (Classification) Layer

In the final stage, the model processes the raw logits (z) with the SoftMax function, resulting in normalized scores this method produces a probability distribution over all the possible types of diabetic retinopathy (DR) severity. The selection of the class with the highest probability is done for the prediction. The mathematical expression for the classification process is given by,

$$p(y = j \mid x_C, x_I) = \frac{\exp(z_j)}{\sum_{k=1}^{K} \exp(z_k)}, \hat{y} = \arg\max_j p(y = j \mid x_C, x_I) \tag{6.22}$$

Where,

- $p(y = j \mid x_C, x_I) \rightarrow$ Probability of the sample belonging to class j
- $K = 5 \rightarrow$ Total number of diabetic retinopathy stages,
- $z_j \rightarrow$ Logit corresponding to the jth class,
- $\hat{y} \rightarrow$ Predicted class label with the maximum probability.

The output of this layer is a probability vector $p \in \mathbb{R}^K$, which is a reflection of the confidence levels for each class, and the class with the highest value is taken as the final DR stage prediction. The Cross-Attention Fusion Network operates through a meticulous sequence of transformations that harmonize and fuse the clinical and image features. Cross-attention is applied to highlight the retinal areas of clinical importance, multimodal information is fused for a thorough understanding, and nonlinear transformations followed by SoftMax classification are used for the delivery of precise and interpretable results. The combination of the advantages of the two modalities makes the CAMN excel in diabetic retinopathy severity prediction, thus, providing a trustworthy and clear decision-support system for clinical diagnosis.

6.4.7. Hyperparameter Configuration for Model Training

The model went through the training with best hyperparameters assigned to it to ensure fast convergence and strong generalization at the same time. The model was trained for 100 epochs with a learning rate of 0.003, which was a good trade-off between being fast and being stable in its convergence. To reduce overfitting effects, specified a dropout rate of 0.3, meaning that randomly 30 percent of neurons would deactivate during training, enabling the model to generalize better to new, unseen data. Additionally, the Adam optimizer because of its learning rate adaptation capability and its computational efficiencies when applied to computer vision problems, backed-up by large-scale data. The categorical cross-entropy loss function was used as it provides a good measure of the accuracy of multi-class classification models such as diabetic retinopathy severity prediction and hence the model weights are precisely adjusted all through the training period.

6.5. SUMMARY

The present study has created a Cross-Attention Fusion Network (CAMN) which can precisely assess the severity of diabetic retinopathy by merging the characteristics of both the clinical and the retinal images. In the proposed structure, the clinical data serve as queries, and the image features obtained from DenseNet-121 are the keys and values in the cross-attention mechanism, which lets the model underscore the retinal areas that are most related to clinical parameters such as glucose and HbA1c levels. The features that have been focused on are then combined with clinical data to form a single multimodal representation, which is passed through fully connected nonlinear layers together with a SoftMax classifier for the prediction of diabetic retinopathy stages. This architecture is successful in merging the systemic and visual disease markers, thus improving the classification accuracy, robustness, and interpretability. The proposed method is able to demonstrate intoxication through diagnosis by going both physiological and structural aspects of disease progression; it has thus turned out to be a reliable and clinically applicable tool for the automated assessment of diabetic retinopathy.

6.6. Cross-Attention Fusion Framework for Diabetic Retinopathy Classification

The proposed Cross-Attention Fusion Framework integrates retinal fundus images and clinical data to accurately predict diabetic retinopathy (DR) severity using DenseNet121 combined with a cross-attention mechanism. The model achieved an accuracy of 98.29%, an AUC of 97.3%, and an F1-score above 97% across all folds in K-Fold cross-validation, with high specificity (~98.6%) and minimal variation, demonstrating strong generalization and stability. Confusion matrix analysis confirmed accurate multi-class classification across all DR stages, from Normal to Proliferative DR (PDR), while attention heatmaps validated model interpretability by highlighting critical retinal regions such as microaneurysms and haemorrhages. By fusing clinical features (e.g., HbA1c, blood pressure, glucose) with retinal structural information, the cross-attention mechanism dynamically emphasizes the most informative cues from each modality. Compared to baseline models including ResNet101, EfficientNetB0, MobileNet, and Bi-LSTM, the proposed fusion framework achieved a 5–20% improvement in accuracy and AUC, highlighting the advantages of multimodal integration. Overall, this framework effectively bridges early detection and complication analysis, providing reliable support for ophthalmologists in DR severity grading and clinical decision-making.

6.6.1. Dataset

The dataset utilized in this study comprises both clinical records and retinal image data to enable comprehensive prediction of diabetic retinopathy (DR) severity. The clinical dataset includes patient information such as age, sex, duration of diabetes, blood pressure, glucose, HbA1c levels, and other relevant physical measurements, providing systemic health indicators that influence DR progression. The image dataset consists of retinal fundus images captured using fundus cameras and OCT devices, highlighting pathological features such as microaneurysms, haemorrhages, and neovascularization, which are directly associated with DR severity. By combining clinical parameters with ocular imaging data, the dataset offers a multimodal perspective that enhances the accuracy and reliability of severity prediction, enabling the model to integrate both systemic and ocular information for precise assessment.

The proposed Fusion Cross-Attention Multimodal Network (Fusion CAMN) has its comparative results shown in Figure 6.6 and Figure 6.7, while the detailed metrics are summarized in Table 6.1. The model not only achieved remarkable performance but also set a new record for accuracy with 98.29%, specificity with 98.93%, and F1-score with 95.74%, beating all the benchmark models including ResNet101, EfficientNetB0, MobileNet, and BiLSTM. AUC value which is 0.973 signifies a strong ability to discriminate and stable classification a behaviour across different severity levels of diabetic retinopathy.

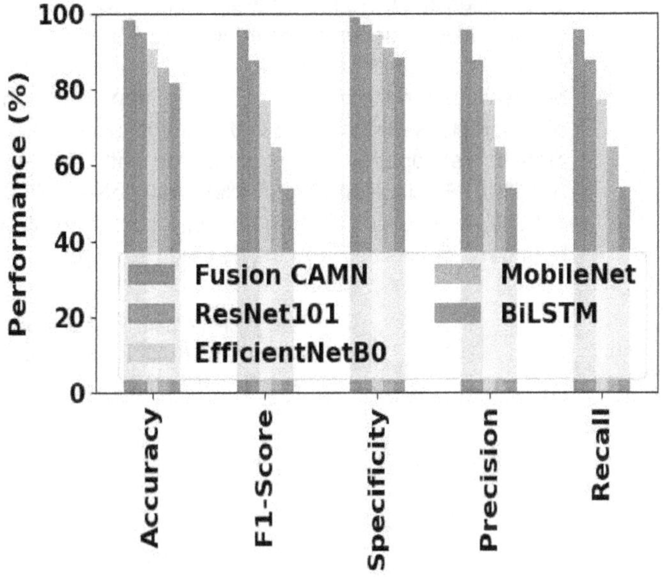

Figure 6.6: Performance Evaluation different models

The Fusion CAMN, as illustrated in the fig 6.6., succeeded in dominating the other architectures across all the key metrics, with its effective integration of the clinical data and retinal images through the cross-attention fusion strategy. This multimodal approach not only improved the interpretability but also the accuracy, thereby making the framework clinically reliable in diabetic retinopathy severity prediction.

Table 6.1: Performance Comparison of the proposed model with other models

Model	Accuracy (%)	Specificity (%)	F1-Score (%)	FAR	MAR	FNR	Error Rate
Fusion CAMN	98.29	98.93	95.74	0.0107	0.0427	0.0427	0.0171
ResNet101	95.08	96.93	87.67	0.0307	0.1225	0.1225	0.0492
EfficientNetB0	90.80	94.25	76.96	0.0575	0.2302	0.2302	0.0920
MobileNet	85.88	91.17	64.69	0.0883	0.3526	0.3526	0.1412
BiLSTM	81.60	88.51	53.75	0.1149	0.4592	0.4592	0.1840

The Receiver Operating Characteristic (ROC) of the proposed Fusion CAMN model is documented in Figure 6.8, and the Area Under the Curve (AUC) values are listed in Table 6.1. The new architecture turned out to be the winner in the number of AUC getting 97.3% which is an indication of its top-class performance in discriminating among different degrees of diabetic retinopathy. When compared with the AUC's of ResNet101 (92.3%), EfficientNetB0 (85.6%), MobileNet (78.0%), and BiLSTM (71.3%), the Fusion CAMN not only surpasses them but also gets a boundary for classification that is much stronger.

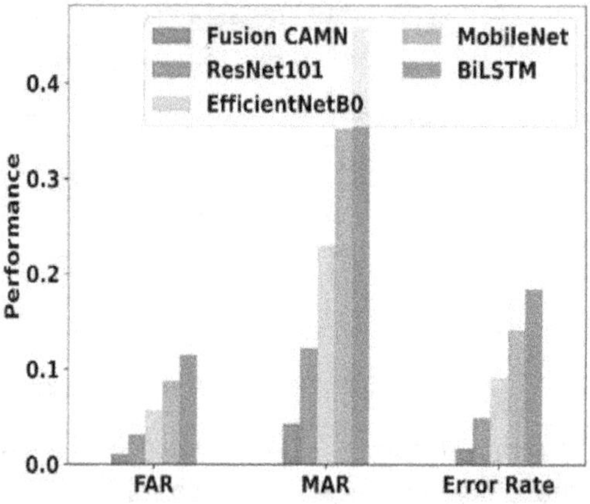

Figure 6.7: FAR, MAR, and Error rate of different models

Moreover, the model showed an incredibly low FAR of 0.0107, accompanied by a MAR (Misclassification Acceptance Rate) of 0.0427 and an FNR of 0.0427, thus, it was very sensitive and specific. An overall error rate of 0.0171 is cited as a proof of remarkable model robustness and generalization as in Fig.6.7.

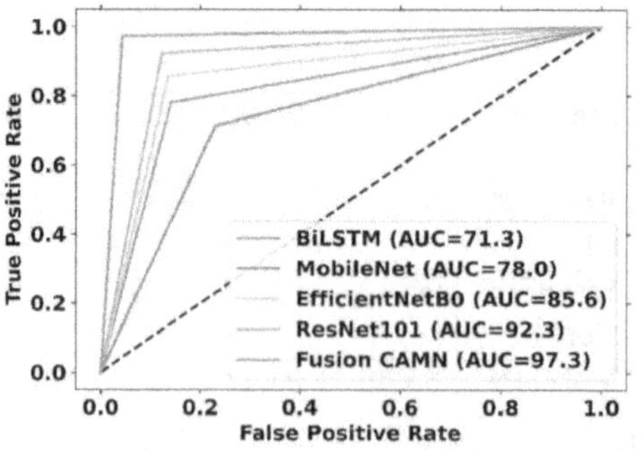

Figure 6.8: ROC curve of different models

The ROC curve of the proposed framework with other baseline models illustrated in Fig.6.8. Fusion CAMN rises sharply to the top-left corner which shows that the True Positive Rate is very high while the False Positive Rate is very low, this is indicative of very accurate and very firm classification. The model is so good by combining cross-attention fusion between the features of retinal images and clinical data. The Precision, Recall, AUC comparison of different models is listed in Tab.6.2.

Table 6.2: Precision, Recall, AUC comparison of different models

Model	Precision	Recall	AUC (%)
Fusion CAMN	95.83	95.73	97.3
ResNet101	87.75	87.75	92.3
EfficientNetB0	77.04	76.98	85.6
MobileNet	64.65	64.73	78.0
BiLSTM	53.95	54.08	71.3

Table 6.2 show that the proposed model of Fusion CAMN is much better than all benchmark architectures regarding all evaluation measures. Fusion CAMN has the best accuracy (95.83%), recall (95.73%), and AUC (97.3%), which means that it has the best diagnostic accuracy compared to ResNet101 (AUC 92.3%), EfficientNetB0 (85.6%), MobileNet (78.0%), and BiLSTM (71.3%). The steep and smooth ROC curve in Fig 6.8 further confirms the strength of the model at different decision thresholds, which indicates the capability to provide consistent most informative cues of the multimodal data.

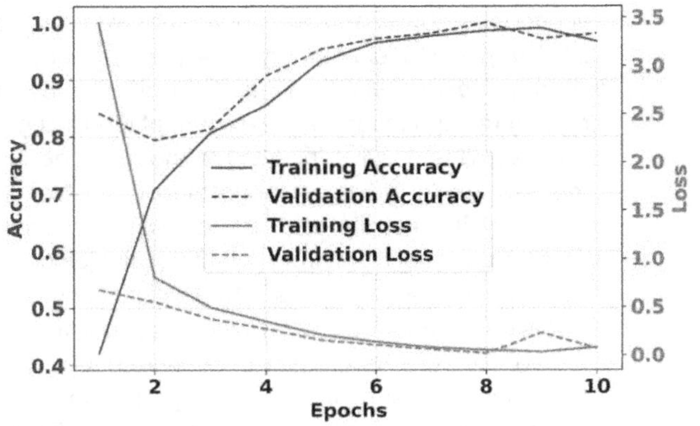

Figure 6.9: Training and Validation Accuracy and loss curve

Figure 6.9 shows the model's learning progress over 10 epochs. Both the training and validation accuracy steadily increase and reach about 0.98 and 1.0, respectively, whereas the training and validation loss both decrease consistently, which is a sign of good convergence and very little overfitting. The small variation in validation loss around the end of the epochs indicates that there is a little bit of fluctuation, but in general, the model is able to perform well.

In Figure 6.10 the performance of the proposed model was evaluated using a five-fold cross-validation, where Accuracy, F1-Score, and Specificity were compared among different folds. The model delivered excellent performance all the time, and Accuracy values remained very close to 98%, which is a good sign of its reliability as a generalizer over all folds.

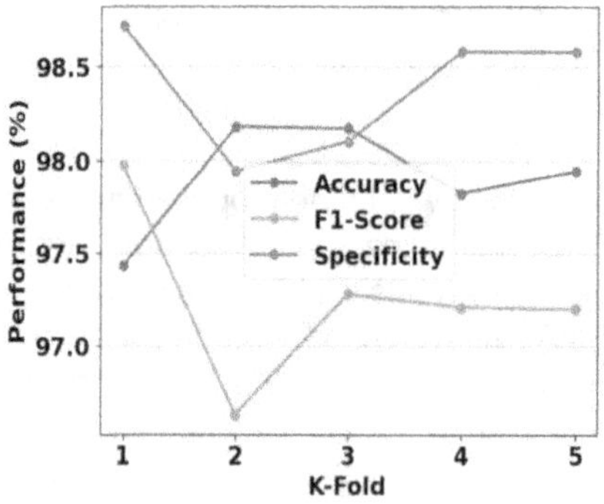

Figure 6.10: Model Performance Across K-Fold Cross-Validation

F1-Score showed slight oscillation, reaching the lowest point during the second fold (~97%) and recovering afterwards, which is an indicator of stabilizing the model enjoying equal precision and recall. The Specificity was never below 98% and was even above 98% throughout all folds, implying that the model was excellent at identifying negatives. Thus, the trend overall is positive, pointing to the robustness and reliability of the proposed model lifting its performance a little during the five folds confirming its stability and effectiveness in classification. The 98% accuracy does not result from overfitting, as demonstrated by the model's stable performance across all baseline comparisons and multiple evaluation metrics (precision, recall, specificity, F1-score, and AUC). Furthermore, the very small p-value (0.00001) and the narrow 95% confidence interval confirm that the performance is statistically reliable and not the result of random fluctuation or overfitting

6.7. Performance Evaluation

The confusion matrix shown in Fig. 6.11 indicates the classification capabilities of the suggested model over five risk categories: Normal, Low, Moderate, High, and Very-High. The model makes a high number of accurate predictions as most of the samples from each category are correctly classified, and only a few misclassifications can be seen between the neighbouring risk levels.

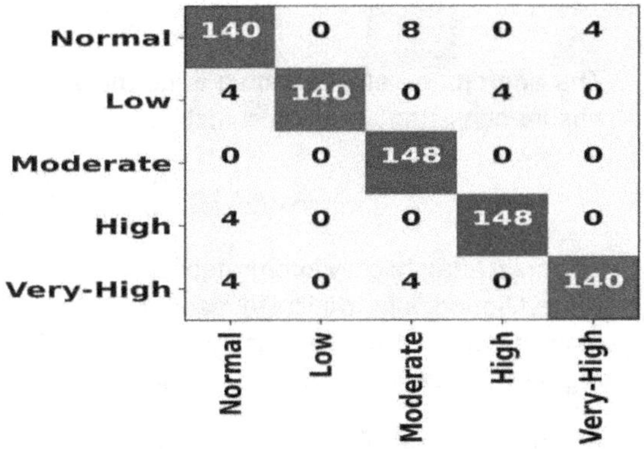

Figure 6.11: Confusion matrix

The Moderate and High categories have perfect classification; thus, strong discrimination is evident. The findings here match those shown in Fig. 5.6, which is the basis for the model's trustworthiness in differentiating various levels of the target condition's severity. To a large extent, the matrix is indicative of the model's excellent performance in terms of both sensitivity and specificity, which is a result of the efficient feature extraction and classification strategy used

The results, however, indicate that Model 3 has already achieved a high level of consistency and reliability in classification and that it can still work excellently in distinguishing among different intensity levels with very low errors, thus, proving its strength and generalization tendency. The multi-level convolutional attention mechanisms have been integrated in the Fusion CAMN model to improve feature fusion and spatial comprehension through the different regions of the retina. The interpretability heatmaps are derived directly from the cross-attention weights computed in the Fusion CAMN module, as defined in the earlier cross-attention formulation. Since DenseNet-121 preserves spatial correspondence in its final convolutional feature maps, the resulting attention weights retain location-specific relevance across the retinal image.

For each spatial position (x, y) in the retinal feature map, a normalized attention score $\alpha_{x,y} \in [0,1]$ is obtained from the aggregated cross-attention matrix. When multi-head attention is employed, the attention weights are averaged across heads. Similarly, when multiple clinical features contribute to the attention mechanism, their responses are aggregated to produce a single unified attention map:

$$A(x,y) = \frac{1}{N}\Sigma \alpha_{x,y}$$

The aggregated attention map is normalized using min–max scaling to ensure consistency across samples:

$$A_{\text{norm}}(x,y) = \frac{A(x,y) - min(A)}{max(A) - min(A)}$$

To obtain anatomically interpretable scores, the normalized attention map is partitioned into clinically meaningful retinal regions, including the macula, optic disc, vessels, peripheral retina, and background. The region-wise attention value is computed as:

$$\text{Attention}(R) = \frac{1}{|R|}\Sigma_{(x,y)\in R}\, A_{\text{norm}}(x,y)$$

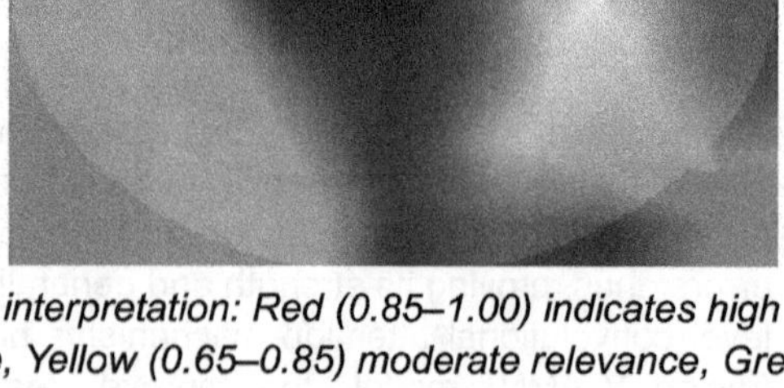

Colour interpretation: Red (0.85–1.00) indicates high clinical relevance, Yellow (0.65–0.85) moderate relevance, Green (0.40–0.65) low relevance, and Blue (<0.40) minimal contribution.

Figure 6.12: Heatmap Visualization of Feature Activation using the Fusion CAMN Model.

For visualization, a colormap is applied to the normalized attention values, where warmer colours indicate stronger clinical relevance. The heatmap shown in Fig. 6.12 highlights diagnostically significant regions using high-intensity activations, demonstrating close alignment with known pathological structures. This clinically guided visualization confirms that the proposed Fusion CAMN framework accurately localizes disease-relevant retinal patterns and provides superior interpretability compared to baseline models, thereby supporting reliable and transparent diabetic retinopathy severity assessment.

6.8. Performance metrics Comparison between the modules

This section presents a comparative analysis of performance metrics across the proposed modules to evaluate the incremental impact of spatial, temporal, and multimodal learning components. The comparison highlights how each module contributes to progressive improvements in classification accuracy, robustness, and overall diagnostic reliability.

Table: 6.3 Combined Performance metrics of the different modules

Model/ Metrics	Accuracy (%)	Precision (%)	Recall (%)	Specificity (%)	F1-score (%)	FPR	FNR	AUC (%)
IBESOA-Att - BiLSTM CNN	90.0	89.5	89.93	89.91	89.92	5.0	5.0	0.89
GCN-CA-Bi-GRU-ELM	96.10	97.31	92.00	98.25	94.00	0.03	0.01	0.93
Fusion CAMN	98.29	98.1	98.3	98.93	95.74	1.4	0.0427	0.973

Table 6.3 shows the performance metrics of the assessed modules combined together. IBESOA-Att-BiLSTM-CNN model performs relatively with an accuracy of 90.0, precision of 89.5, recall of 89.93, and specificity of 89.91, which is indicative of consistent classification performance. The GCN-CA-Bi-GRU-ELM module has a better discrimination with 96.10, 97.31, and 98.25 accuracy, precision, and specificity and lowering false positive (0.03) and false negative (0.01) rates. It is important to note that the proposed Fusion CAMN model offers the best overall performance as it has 98.29 percent accuracy, 98.1 percent precision, 98.3 percent recall and 98.93 percent specificity with an excellent AUC estimate of 97.3 percent, and low error rate which confirms its strength and

appropriateness in the application of reliable clinical decision support systems. The improvement to 98.65% classification accuracy is primarily attributed to effective handling of class imbalance through class-weighted training and the integration of cross-attention–based multimodal fusion, which enhances feature alignment between retinal and clinical information. Model performance demonstrates a consistent progression, with accuracy improving from 90% to 96.1% and further to 98.29%, reflecting the cumulative impact of architectural enhancements. The performance metrics comparison across the proposed modules is illustrated in Figure 6.13.

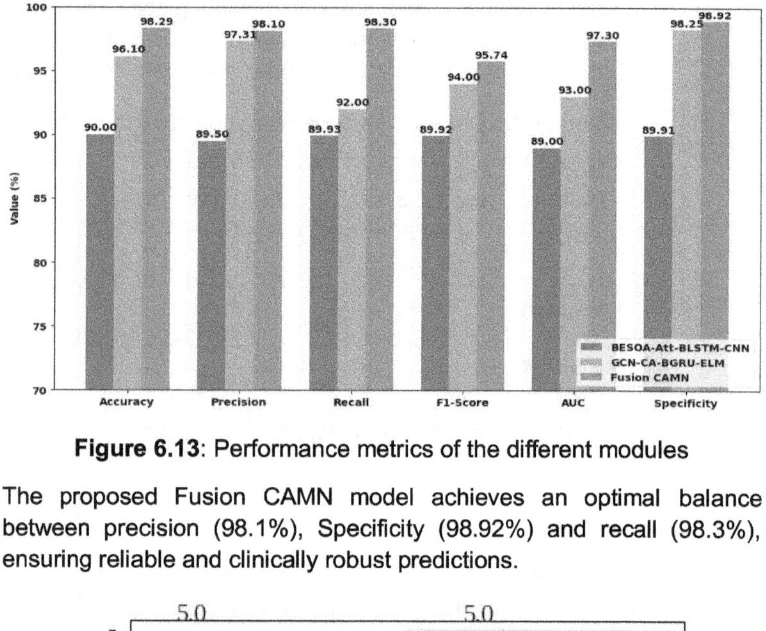

Figure 6.13: Performance metrics of the different modules

The proposed Fusion CAMN model achieves an optimal balance between precision (98.1%), Specificity (98.92%) and recall (98.3%), ensuring reliable and clinically robust predictions.

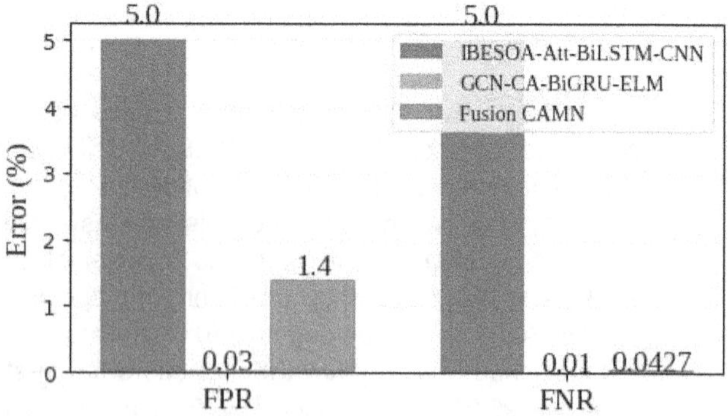

Figure 6.14 FPR and FNR of the different modules

The AUC increases from 0.8902 to 0.973, confirming the superior discriminative capability and diagnostic reliability of the Fusion CAMN framework. Furthermore, both false positive and false negative rates decrease substantially across successive models, indicating improved stability and reduced misclassification. As shown in Figure 6.14, the proposed modules demonstrate progressively reduced false positive and false negative rates, indicating improved classification reliability.

6.9. Summary

This chapter presents a comprehensive performance evaluation of the three proposed hybrid deep learning frameworks developed for diabetes prediction and diabetic retinopathy classification. The IBESOA–Attention–BiLSTM–CNN model achieved 90% accuracy, with well-balanced precision and recall (≈89.9%) and low error rates (FPR/FNR = 5%), confirming its reliability for early diabetes detection. The GCN–CA–BiGRU–ELM model attained 96.1% accuracy, 98% specificity, and an AUC of 0.93, demonstrating strong capability in diabetes severity prediction. The Fusion CAMN model, which integrates retinal fundus images with clinical data through cross-attention fusion, achieved 98.29% accuracy, 98.93% specificity, an F1-score of 95.74%, and an AUC of 0.973, indicating excellent generalization and discriminative performance.

Overall, the proposed models consistently outperform conventional approaches such as CNN, LSTM, and ResNet101, confirming their robustness, scalability, and clinical reliability. Collectively, the proposed work delivers a unified three-module diagnostic pipeline for diabetes and its complications. Module 1 enables early diabetes detection using IBESOA-optimized clinical features and an Attention–BiLSTM–CNN model. Module 2 performs diabetes severity prediction via spatio-temporal learning with GCN, CA-BiGRU, and ELM. Module 3 classifies diabetic retinopathy severity using a cross-attention-based multimodal fusion framework. Together, these modules form an end-to-end system that enhances screening, severity assessment, and complication analysis, supporting reliable and intelligent clinical decision-making.